Compassionate Relational Therapy

Weaving together known successful interventions with innovative and new methods, Compassionate Relational Therapy (CRT) offers a unique and cohesive method to strengthen relationships through decreased judgment and increased compassion within the self and with others.

Integrating evidence-based practices of family systems theory, compassion-focused therapy, and mindful self-compassion, CRT reframes and expands existing approaches to better fit the needs of romantic and familial relationship therapy. This model examines interaction and communication patterns to unfold and release guilt and shame with compassion and nonjudgmental curiosity toward our assumptions or unmet needs. With applications for family therapy, romantic therapy, and sex therapy, readers will learn the skills to move clients toward self-kindness, situational and bodily mindfulness, and compassion toward a loved one's humanness, to create a sense of relational safety and connection without dependence. This book includes CRT's core theory of change, guides for all stages of treatment, and interventions unique to this model that can also be integrated into existing models of therapy. Additionally, it offers new interventions such as compassionate contextualization, temporary agreements, and compassionate restorations for work with diverse populations, with example cases and conversations in each chapter for easy application.

Written in a compassionate and accessible style, this is an essential guide for mental health clinicians of all kinds and all experience levels, from students to seasoned professionals.

Bethany Suppes, PhD, LMFT, is an AAMFT-Approved Supervisor. She is the author of *Family Systems Theory Simplified* along with other publications and presentations regarding compassion- and systemic-based supervision and therapeutic practices. She currently runs a private practice, serves as Chief of Curriculum Development at TwoX Labs (a continuing education provider), and is a board member of the Washington Association of Marriage and Family Therapy.

Emma Christie-Foster, MA, LMFT, is a marriage and family therapist and sex therapist with extensive clinical and research experience in compassion-based approaches and therapeutic practices. She currently runs a private practice where she specializes in sex therapy and works with individuals and couples.

Compassionate Relational Therapy

Core Concepts and Applications

Bethany Suppes and Emma Christie-Foster

Routledge
Taylor & Francis Group

NEW YORK AND LONDON

Designed cover image: Getty Images

First published 2026
by Routledge
605 Third Avenue, New York, NY 10158

and by Routledge
4 Park Square, Milton Park, Abingdon, Oxon, OX14 4RN

Routledge is an imprint of the Taylor & Francis Group, an informa business

© 2026 Bethany Suppes and Emma Christie-Foster

ISBN: 978-1-032-85570-7 (hbk)
ISBN: 978-1-032-84891-4 (pbk)
ISBN: 978-1-003-51873-0 (ebk)

DOI: 10.4324/9781003518730

Typeset in Sabon
by Apex CoVantage, LLC

We dedicate this text to the clinicians and professionals who seek to lean into compassion with ourselves, our loved ones, and our patients, even when it is countercultural to do so.

Contents

Preface: A Letter to Our Readers

Dearest Colleague,

As therapists, we get to have a pretty wonderful job. We get to enter the lives of those around us in an intimate and open way. We bear witness to the most heart-wrenching stories and are audience to beautiful moments of reconciliation. We receive tales of tragedy and heartbreak and can hold hope for them when it feels like they have none. We hear stories of suffering, even interwoven with joy. We walk alongside people in a space that can feel sacred, and when our time with them is through, we are left with the memory that can feel akin to a sense of loss. They are not our friends and really never can be, yet we find ourselves knowing intimate details about their lives, their hopes, their failures, and their triumphs. In ways, the inspiration for this book began with these relationships with clients.

When we first enter school to study to be a counselor or therapist, we embark on a journey of self-growth. We learn about aspects of our personalities, parts of life that feel challenging, or even meet parts of ourselves we didn't realize had such an impact on our worldviews or selves. Lucky for us, this self-exploration never stops in our field of work. While we help others cope and grow, we also learn to cope and grow differently ourselves. No matter how seasoned a therapist you may be, it is amazing what we can continue to find and learn within ourselves. This feels important to recognize because this perspective of being a lifelong learner is not exclusive to education; it includes learning how we understand and relate to the world we are in. As of writing this preface in early 2025, many people are feeling a strong sense of tension in that relationship – that is to say, we might not like the world much right now.

Not long ago, when working with a client, we landed on the phrase, "In a world full of bigotry and weaponized fear, compassion is the new counterculture." That phrase has stuck with us ever since. we've been applying compassionate concepts into our therapeutic work for years, but that was the phrase that encapsulated why in a way that seemed so beautiful and so needed. And what better space for people to explore that countercultural movement, both in themselves and their relationships, than in the safety of therapy?

We authored this manuscript as two individuals who have benefited greatly from the practice of compassion for self and others. As two people who enjoy research (maybe more than the average person), we wanted to explore more deeply what compassion can look like in the therapeutic context, particularly from our systemic lens as marriage and family therapists. Way back in 2019, Bethany's doctoral dissertation focused on the impact of self-compassion-oriented therapy to romantic relationship satisfaction for women. Likely to no one's surprise, the outcome showed a consistent benefit! What surprised us more was the lack of research about therapeutic interventions rooted in compassion aimed for relationships, either families and romantic relationships! Personally and professionally, we feel deeply that compassion is a central factor in the therapeutic experience. Great change and growth can occur where there is both an absence of judgment and active presence of kindness and mindfulness. From that belief grew the initial constructs of Compassionate Relational Therapy (CRT).

This text aims to provide an overview for those interested in integrating compassion-based interventions and ideas into working with relationships. You may also find, as you read, that age-old applicability to your own life. Honestly, we hope you do! We hope you reflect on how compassion is present and can be nurtured in your relationships and your wellbeing.

Furthermore, we hope to equip clinicians with tools and language solely oriented in compassion, providing a new means to explore challenges and trials that embraces both emotion and cognitive contributions to change. We aren't trying to reinvent the therapeutic wheel. We use and scaffold off successful ideas and interventions with the new layer of emphasis on decreasing felt shame, replacing it with authentic compassion. But we're getting ahead of ourselves!

In an effort to be transparent, open, and authentic, we both included stories from our own lives sprinkled throughout the chapters. These include our own memories, client experiences, and personal thoughts along the way. Many chapters also include case examples showing the application of CRT interventions. All case studies included in the book are based on real situations or client accounts with identifiable information and details changed to protect their confidentiality. For the sake of content clarity (and brevity), information and session details have been reduced, and our descriptions may show a more abbreviated "screenshot" version of what interventions look like in the therapy sessions.

Last but not least, in writing this book, we recognize our privilege as two cisgendered white women with multiple graduate degrees between the two of us living relatively comfortably in the United States. These positions of privilege have undeniably impacted our experience both in our world-views and as therapists. We have done our best to design a therapy models that remains relevant and available to a multitude of audiences, including intentionality toward inclusivity of diverse identities, experiences, and equity of care. Of course, there is always more work to be done in pursuit of allyship and representation. That's not an insult to us; that is putting our theory into practice.

We believe not only in this material but in the change, connection, healing, and restoration that compassion can bring. We have lived and continue to live this with friends, family, and clients. We hope you find this text to be compelling, informative, and experientially reflective. We look forward to continuing to discover more about the infinite applications of compassion to improve quality of life right alongside you!

Authentically and sincerely,
Bethany and Emma

Part I

Theoretical Foundations

Chapter 1

Self-Compassion and Compassion-Based Therapies

A Launching Point

Right off the cuff, concepts like compassion and self-compassion bring with them an imagery of softness, like fluffy clouds and cozy blankets. While these qualities are true, the simile leaves gaps for misconceptions of compassion, like believing it lacks depth or dismisses accountability. Fortunately, compassion is so much more than that. Compassion has been part of conversations in self-help and psychotherapy for a few decades now, yet there has not been an approach that specifically focuses on using compassion to create meaningful change in relationships. We are here to change that.

This chapter identifies the concepts and benefits of compassion and self-compassion, how they have been addressed therapeutically so far, and their personal and interpersonal benefits. We will then summarize the limitations of other approaches in treating relationship issues.

What is Compassion?

Compassion is both the intimate awareness of suffering (one's own and others') and the desire to relieve it. It is the feeling *for* a person's experience and perspective, and the subsequent motivation to engage in change. Toward other people, it is a desire to meet someone where they are at and attune to their suffering without taking it on as our own. Compassion has roots in Buddhist philosophy and positive psychology. It assumes suffering is inescapable, but the extent of suffering depends on a person's resiliency. By accepting the present for all that it is, including people's roles in it, compassion builds resilience.

What is Self-Compassion?

Kristin Neff, the pioneer of the modern understanding of self-compassion, beautifully describes self-compassion as the process of turning compassion inward. Self-compassion is being open to one's own suffering and hurt, not

DOI: 10.4324/9781003518730-2

avoiding or disconnecting. Self-compassion offers nonjudgmental under-standing toward our pain, inadequacies, and failures as part of the human experience. It generates the desire to alleviate one's suffering and to heal oneself through kindness, not criticism. Self-compassion, therefore, is more than behavioral self-care. It is opening ourselves up to feel both the joys and peace of life along with discomfort and pain, instead of ignoring or attempting to push it down or bury it in a teeny tiny double locked box in our hearts or minds. Neff's description of self-compassion, including its three tenets, has been inspirational and hugely impactful in our lives per-sonally and therapeutically.

Tenets of Self-Compassion

Self-compassion is a triad of equally valuable attributes: self-kindness, shared humanity, and mindfulness. These three components are inter-related: self-kindness is part of mindfulness, part of connecting to one's humanity, and vice versa.

1. Self-Kindness

Simply defined, self-kindness is the capacity to offer ourselves gentle real-ism without judgment or personalization. It is the golden rule in reverse, treating ourselves with the kindness and understanding we often offer oth-ers in challenging times. Self-kindness is being a friend to oneself and com-forting ourselves like a friend would through care and support. This offers emotional and physical gentleness with yourself. Self-compassion improves one's ability and comfort to be compassionate and kind toward others, too. The learning curve can be to figure out how to give this to ourselves even though we might feel as though we don't deserve it, and getting to a point where we believe that we do.

Self-kindness is juxtaposed by self-judgment. Self-judgment is the prod-uct of self-criticism and shame. Self-judgment breeds anger, shame, and blame when life doesn't go as we hoped. Self-judgment tends to belittle, reject, or minimize one's suffering, even condemn a person's character as a result of that suffering. This harsh perspective leads to higher levels of stress and emotional reactivity; in those moments, kindness is exactly what we all need.

2. Shared Humanity

Shared or common humanity is the reminder that suffering is a common human experience. Everyone is likely to experience feelings of inadequacy, self-doubt, disappointment, and pain at some point in life. To say such is not a comparison ("Other people have had it worse"). Instead, shared humanness acknowledges how suffering is a part of life: "My pain is unique, and I am not alone in it." This is considered the feature that differentiates self-compassion from simple self-acceptance or self-love, which lack communal context.

The inverse of feeling connected to other people is feeling isolated. Isolation is the belief that we are alone in our suffering or the only one who has to "deal with something like this." However, a fact of life is that we all suffer, and comparison to how one person suffers differently from someone else is unhelpful and dismissive. At one point, one way or another, every human will experience suffering and hardship. To experience this is not indicative of personal failure or an unforgivable flaw. To quote Captain Jean-Luc Picard, "It is possible to commit no mistakes and still lose. That is not weakness. That is life."

3. Mindfulness

Mindfulness is the capacity to see situations for what they are with a more neutral, non-personalized perspective. This part of self-compassion focuses on approaching our negative emotions and feelings with balance, an equilibrative stance, and in context. It is like a camera lens that can zoom in to focus on details but can also zoom out to see more of what's around us. The goal is to navigate thoughts and feelings so that they are neither dramatized and over-exaggerated nor muted and suppressed. Ultimately, mindfulness is both a process and outcome; it is something you both practice and achieve.

The antithesis of mindfulness is over-identification. Over-identification is the irrational assumption of being responsible for or in control of events or ideas outside yourself. Over-identification overlaps with cognitive distortions such as personalizing, ruminating, magnification and minimization, should statements, all-or-nothing thinking, and mind-reading or jumping to conclusions. It is through mindfulness that we learn to compassionately challenge even these stubborn sides of ourselves.

Myths About Self-Compassion

Unfortunately, as with all well-intentioned things, there are ways to misinterpret self-compassion, resulting in numerous myths about its construct and purpose. Here are five common misconceptions about compassion and self-compassion:

- "Self-compassion is the same as self-pity."
- "Self-compassion is a form of weakness."

- "Self-compassion invites complacency."
- "Self-compassion encourages self-centeredness."
- "Self-compassion is selfish."

To be clear, these are untrue. These misconceptions come from a belief that if we aren't actively harsh with ourselves, we risk becoming morally complacent and egotistical. To the contrary, self-compassion has been shown to be a greater force of motivation than self-punishment.

> **A Note from Bethany:** At one point in my life, I wanted to be a runner. I signed up to run my first 5k and started to train. At first, I was harsh with myself. I thought, "Why aren't you going faster? You're out of breath already? Really?" It didn't make the next steps any easier. Race day came, and as I was losing steam in the last bit, I heard people along the path clapping and saying things like, "You're almost there! You've got this!" and, "Great job!" In that moment it clicked: Those were the messages that gave me my second (or third or fourth) wind that actually enabled me to succeed, not harshness or criticism.

Self-compassion and self-affirmation actually build one another up to increase forms of efficiency and effectiveness. Self-compassion is not passive; research repeatedly endorses self-compassion as one of the most resilient forms of coping possible! Unlike the extrinsic measures of self-esteem, self-compassion accepts a person's flaws without dooming an individual for having them. Let's talk about that.

Compassion Versus Empathy and Esteem

A common misconception about compassion is that it is interchangeable with empathy or esteem. Maybe this could be considered the sixth myth. However, they are actually very different physiologically, emotionally, and mentally. We defined compassion as being understanding and open to the inevitable experience of suffering, not avoiding or disconnecting from it, and finding the gentle motivation to heal mindfully. Here's how empathy and esteem differ:

Empathy

Empathy is the attempt to put ourselves in someone else's perspective to consider their feelings, thoughts, and choices. This visceral attempt, however, remains stuck in one's own emotional position: "This is how *I* would feel if I was in that position." Compassion, on the other hand, seeks to understand the other person's feelings without having to relate or reach the same emotional stance. Empathy can be well-intentioned and a useful early step toward compassion; through it, we demonstrate that we are listening and aligning with another person. Empathy is often discussed as a fundamental tool for successful therapy for this reason, assuming empathic connection creates a bond that makes the individual feel cared for and heard. However, untethered empathy can be like emotional quicksand; it is easier to be pulled in than out. It makes space for vicarious distress through overidentifying with someone else's suffering. Empathy is compassion without adequate boundaries. Ultimately, it makes it much more difficult to then be emotionally available for others in our lives, including ourselves.

Esteem

Esteem is a measured value of one's contributions to a relationship, situation, or outcome. Self-esteem places one's value on how a person contributes to those or achieves external goals. Esteem can also be assessed from a social constructionist lens. This method determines how valuable something – or someone – is based on how this compares to the perceived value of others' contributions. That is to say, a person's worth may seem dependent on how valuable their contributions are to the world, a relationship, or a conversation. Sounds pretty subjective, right? Unfortunately, self-esteem generally requires external evidence of one's contributions, especially outcomes. Not only that, the goalpost that defines success frequently moves as soon as you meet it, leading to a lack of the craved external validation that warrants higher self-esteem. Research shows both high and low self-esteem are associated with distorted self-knowledge, but only low self-compassion perpetuates the same.

Self-compassion and seeking self-wellness does not require comparison to others. Good self-esteem can depend on good times or self-deceit; self-compassion, on the other hand, endures with hope and kindness. To use a sports metaphor, where esteem is a fair-weather fan, self-compassion is the thirteenth man.

Benefits of Self-Compassion

Self-compassion can play a crucial role in the psychological and physical wellbeing of a person and their quality of life. For example, self-compassion can offer physical health benefits including boosting immune system functionality, and mindfulness is positively correlated with improving sleep. Additionally, research has demonstrated self-compassion to mediate overall mental health. Self-compassionate people tend to be happier, more creative, have a strong value system, and feel more comfortable expressing themselves. Self-compassion has an overall positive correlation with life satisfaction, particularly when mediated specifically by the presence of hope. Here are just a few ways that self-compassion has been shown to improve life quality:

1. Decreasing Anxiety and Depression

Self-compassion has repeatedly demonstrated effectiveness at treating anxiety and its symptoms, even more so than self-esteem. Self-compassion, especially mindfulness, positively correlates to ambiguity tolerance and stress resilience, such as decreased feelings of overwhelm with goal-directed activities and lowered levels of anticipatory anxiety. Self-compassion has been shown to perpetuate a more rational, less obsessive outlook on difficult life experiences and implementation of healthier coping skills. Self-compassion negatively correlates with procrastination, perfectionism, fear of being outperformed or making mistakes, or tying achievement with self-worth – all attributes associated with low motivation. Greater self-compassion positively correlates with persistence in tasks, willingness to seek help, enjoyment, self-control, stress management, and setting attainable goals.

2. Increasing Emotional Regulation

Higher self-compassion is positively associated with higher emotional regulation, decreased reactivity, and improvement in adaptive psychological functioning. Adaptive psychological functioning includes effective coping methods, greater sense of hope and resilience or hardiness, less ineffectiveness, and decreased presence of interpersonal distrust. Mindfulness aids in emotional regulation via compassionate validation of emotions, practicing self-reflection, learning effective communication, and celebrating successes. In the popular Five Factor Model, mindfulness positively correlates with psychological wellbeing, agreeability, extraversion, openness, and conscientiousness. It negatively correlates to neuroticism, which is typically associated with emotion regulation, especially anxiety and depression. The practice of accepting negative emotion has been shown to positively affect mental illnesses such as borderline personality disorder and eating disorders. Self-compassion predicts one's emotional regulation capacity more than risk factors such as presence or severity of childhood trauma, maltreatment or addiction history, and current psychological distress.

3. Improved Interpersonal Relationships

Research shows the presence of compassion offers numerous benefits to interpersonal relationships of all kinds. Compassion improves social connectedness, such as appropriate boundary setting, increases acceptance of feedback from others with decreased rumination on self-image, decreased likelihood to people-please. It also helps to see others' perspectives, communicate effectively, and demonstrate altruism and forgiveness for self and others. Mindfulness, specifically, has positive correlation with empathic concern, relational satisfaction, and perspective-taking. This increases relational peace through intentional focus on positive experiences and emotions in the relationship and improved balanced reflection on one's own thoughts, feelings, strengths, and weaknesses. Compassion uniquely maintains sensitivity to context, individual differences, and improved ability to give and receive support and accountability. These thoughtful interactions result in more constructive problem-solving and reduce villainization of one another.

4. Improved Romantic Relationships

The presence of self-compassion in a romantic relationship benefits romantic relationship satisfaction. Self-compassion aids the meeting of individual needs for autonomy, competence, and communication that are essential to relationship well-being. Additionally, self-compassion regulates perception of problem severity and efficacy. That is to say, even when the problem does not change or resolve, the perspective of suffering shifts, thanks to self-compassion. Individuals with higher self-compassion are more likely to offer kindness to themselves and their partners, such as improved ability to identify healthy behavior in their romantic relationships such as respect, support, and autonomy. Conversely, low levels of compassion results in more detached, controlling, and self-critical thoughts, feelings, and behaviors that block relationship intimacy.

Though not directly labeled as compassion, several relationship qualities align with the skill and benefit of it. Couples who experience deep, intimate, emotional connection are usually more successful, positive, and happy compared to those without that intimate support. People in more satisfied relationships tend to evenly give and receive support from their partners, finding fulfillment without minimizing one's needs in favor of compromise. Similarly, satisfying relationships tend to encompass more constructive conflict, using a tone of gentle curiosity and compassionate acceptance. Emotional regulation helps us be more receptive to a partner's humor, creativity, problem-solving, empathy, and non-defensive listening.

All this research comes together to consistently show the benefits of compassion and self-compassion both personally and relationally. Therefore it is unsurprising that a therapeutic modality would be designed aiming to increase such.

Compassion in Therapy

Research has shown that compassion is natural and can be heightened with effort and practice, including through clinical intervention. With time and intentionality, compassionate language becomes more automatic, even in hard times. However, compassion-based therapies are not limited to changing perspective on past events or current behaviors; they have the intention to shift worldview long term. Compassion-based therapies are open for diverse clientele due to it being more mindful- and emotion-driven than cognitive. These techniques have demonstrated significant outcomes working with anxiety; depression; psychosis; trauma survivors; eating disorders, including full cessation of symptoms; personality disorders, including at a one-year follow-up; and with mental health professionals' own stress management. As of the writing of this text, there are two prominent compassion-based therapies: Compassion-Focused Therapy and Compassionate Mindfulness Training.

Compassion-Focused Therapy (CFT)

Developed by Paul Gilbert, Compassion-Focused Therapy (CFT) is designed for individuals and groups. It looks to change means of self-correction from critical harshness to kindness, felt safety, and warmth toward oneself and others. In theory, shifting away from self-blame and condemnation creates space for receptivity to efforts to cope with life's challenges. CFT works to objectively reflect on one's values, behaviors, thoughts, and emotions, inviting kinder understanding to the parts of oneself one has previously shamed or called unacceptable. It does this through a three-system model: threat detection/protection; drive and resource seeking; soothing, rest, and connection. Per the modality, healing occurs as people learn to transition between them with nonjudgmental reflection and work toward congruence among them. Participants start by neutralizing any dominant self-criticism, perceived isolation, or over-identification and correcting any misperceptions about compassion, as identified above. Progressively, CFT aids individuals to develop compassion through a cycle of offering compassion for self, offering compassion for others, and receiving compassion from others.

CFT incorporates psychoeducation about compassion fatigue and affect-regulation methods along with normalizing; talking to oneself as a friend; identification of context within oneself; self-soothing methods such as slow, deep breathing; nonjudgmental identification of unhelpful coping strategies; introduction of mindfulness practices and meditation; and imagery techniques and safe place identification. This model integrates easily into other therapeutic models because it agrees with core concepts of self-initiated change through change of thoughts, behaviors, or emotions. It can also stand alone as a course focusing primarily on emotional and behavioral self-regulation.

Compassionate Mindfulness Training (CMT)

Compared to CFT, Compassionate Mindfulness Training (CMT) places more emphasis on one specific concept of self-compassion. CMT was designed by Kristin Neff, who is the founding theorist, of sorts, for self-compassion-based self-improvement. With Christopher Germer, Neff designed CMT for those with high self-criticism and shame to teach self-soothing and self-reassuring. CMT believes the solution is not to be rid of the self-critic but instead to offer it the love and acceptance it craves. The training's design is based on key attributes and skills of self-care and compassion: care for wellbeing, sensitivity to distress, sympathy, distress tolerance, empathy, and nonjudgment, with the skills of attention, reasoning, behavior, sensory, feeling, and imagery.

CMT demonstrates therapeutic benefit coping with feelings of inferiority, submissive behavior, and shame and numerous psychological disorders. This difference could impact an individual's ability to manage negative affect. This mirrors multiple studies' findings of decreased self-judgment, though without statistically significant change in interpersonal reactivity or compassion toward others. CMT is most commonly used is a group setting with experiential integration for three, six, or eight sessions.

Compassion-Based Therapies Treating Relationships

Improving self-compassion, including through therapeutic intervention, has been shown to improve romantic relationship satisfaction based on shifts in expectations and acceptance of the present. Compassion-based therapies can be integrated with other emotion-based therapies because they consistently utilize nurturing language. They can lean into coregulation and secure attachment aided by self-soothing skills to ease dysregulation in session or mid-conflict.

Overall, CFT has been used to help individuals and by proxy help relationships. CFT helps clients be more accepting of human imperfections and limitations and increases willingness to compromise. Conversely, low levels of self-compassion align with being more detached and controlling in romantic relationships and self-critical to the point of blocking intimacy. However, the direct application of CFT to treat romantic relationships or work with families remains minimal. A version of the model, Compassion-Focused Positive Couple Therapy (CFPCT), is vaguely referenced in an article that focuses on narcissistic men, but is otherwise nonexistent. It describes intentional emphasis on identifying and cultivating positive emotions, experiences, and qualities in relationship and increasing awareness of how one's thoughts, feelings, and behaviors impact one's partner. However, beyond this general description, there is no specified information regarding interventions or theory of change beyond endorsing roots in CFT.

CMT's program is built to focus on individuals, but it is possible for multiple members of a family or intimate partnership to participate in a group together. Like couples counseling, mindfulness positively correlates with effective communication, emotional regulation, problem resolution, relationship satisfaction and wellbeing, skilled responses in relationship distress, and empathy and acceptance between partners with decreased emotional reactivity or presence of negative behaviors. These results were most prominent when the mindfulness training was completed by the couple together rather than individually, though it can be helpful either way.

A lesser-known approach utilizing compassion in couples therapy is Cognitively-Based Compassion Training for Couples (CBCT-fC), which is described as intending to be more preventative than a therapeutic treatment. This modality describes six modules, or steps, over two phases focusing on self- and other/coregulation. These modules move from focused, slow breathing to clear the mind, nurturing an inner observer that is more detached and neutral, fostering self-compassion, building empathic reflection skills for others, emphasis on interconnectedness, and ultimately fostering compassion toward others, specifically a partner, with attention to aiding in decreasing their suffering. Like CFT and MSC, this approach is described in research as provided more often in a group structure, not couples therapy.

Lastly, the Child and Family Institute based in northeast United States designed a therapeutic method called Compassion-Focused Parent Therapy (CFPT). This approach integrates attributes of numerous therapeutic models and focuses on removing blaming language toward parents that can come from a child being the identified patient in therapy. Per their website, "CFPT understands that each parent brings their own psychological and cultural histories, including intergenerational trauma, into the therapy room which is deeply connected to their personal views on parenting, their strengths and limitations as a parent," all of which impact their ability to receive and implement new parenting techniques. They utilize radical compassion and collaborative problem-solving to support parental skill-building that remains compassion-based. This approach is likely most similar to the work proposed in this text, particularly the lens of the therapist's role to exemplify the compassionate skills we hope to enrich in clients.

Strengths of Current Compassion-Based Therapies

Compassion-based therapies focus on the importance of building individuals' capacity to access, tolerate, and direct their emotions mindfully. It cultivates a way to help people better navigate the complexities of our thoughts, emotions, and feelings that are more prosocial and healthy. These modalities do well conceptualizing a problem with a balance of internal and external awareness, which aids in realistic reflection of how change can occur. They emphasize the roles of validation and self-love in motivating behavioral change, offering means to balance kindness and accountability to create change. This is particularly important in the unique compassion-driven focus on decreasing shame. Research analyzing CFT and CMT demonstrate meaningful change both during and after therapy treatment. Additional longitudinal research has shown long-term improved self-compassion and life satisfaction contribute to overall improved quality of life. This includes decreasing stress and depression, and increasing resilience, gratitude, and curiosity both during and after the interventions.

Limits of Existing Compassion-Based Therapies

Despite an exponential growth in academic publications regarding self-compassion over the past two decades, the approaches remain limited. The practices remain focused on individual and group therapy applications. As previously said, applications to couples has been predominantly described as co-occurring individual therapy that both members of the couple are present for; at best, providing communication scripts. Additionally, research and approaches surrounding compassion and self-compassion currently lack attentiveness to sociocultural influence on self-compassion. Lastly, while there is abundant and recurring valid and reliable evidence supporting compassion-based therapies, these outcomes have not consistently been found as statistically significant. There is also some concern that the self-reports may not be reliable, leaning into possible people-pleasing tendencies, especially if the individual has not experienced compassion previously at critical moments in life.

Conclusion

Compassion, distinct from esteem or empathy, emphasizes loving self and others. Compassion and self-compassion have been proven repeatedly to benefit relational wellbeing, and research shows abundantly the benefits of increasing compassion through therapeutic means. It is a skill that can be developed in clinical contexts. Historically, these clinical settings have been rooted in individual and group therapies. We have begun to recognize that increasing compassion relationally, for romantic partners or for family, can drastically improve those relationships as well. CFT has laid a wonderful groundwork and established that compassion thrives best when multidirectional – given and received – in relationships. However, existing approaches miss one big variable: The relationship itself. We have designed Compassionate Relational Therapy specifically to address this key shortcoming, integrating the underlying beliefs and skills of compassion-based therapies with the relational and systemic communication and interaction considerations of family systems theory.

Chapter 2

Family Systems Theory

A Primer for Compassion

Despite its name, family systems theory (FST) could be described as a theory of human interaction, not just families. The same could be said of Compassionate Relational Therapy (CRT). It identifies patterns in how we interact with our fellow humans in the workplace, in school, in the grocery store, at the doctor's office, in the government – everything!

FST looks at relationship dynamics and what influences those. It is more than awareness that relationships and upbringing impact someone along with their biology, and it's not a debate of which is more influential (nature versus nurture). This chapter provides a summary of FST's foundations and contribution to the therapy field; it will then cover the core concepts of the theory. Chief of these is the postmodern role of personal context (how we relate ourselves to the world), a central idea in CRT, too.

What is Family Systems Theory?

FST is the application of general systems theory to humans, highlighting how the relationship between individuals contributes to functionality and outcomes as much as the individuals themselves. These relationships – and the individuals in them – are called systems. Systems are interrelated units bound together by shared qualities, such as, of course, families. However, as is commonly said among FST therapists, "the whole is greater than the sum of its parts." Systems are more than the individual contributions of the people in them; the relationships themselves are factors in functionality. Metaphorically, it is comparable to literature being more than a sequence of letters and music being more than a series of notes.

Cybernetics is also a central component of FST. First-order cybernetics propose that an observer can be purely objective, an outsider watching without influencing. Second-order cybernetics, on the other hand, asserts that even without direct interaction, an observer influences the observed simply by being there. Observers are also influenced by what they observe.

DOI: 10.4324/9781003518730-3

People are innately part of systems and exchange influence. People influence a context and the context influences them, perpetually.

For example, let's say you walk into a store and the employee, formerly alone in the space, is dancing to the music over the speakers. Without saying anything, you observe this behavior. However, simply by becoming aware that you are there, the employee may stop dancing. Being aware of being observed changes behavior.

The commonly used comparison distinguishing these cybernetic types is a thermometer (first-order) versus a thermostat (second-order). While a thermometer can only read the temperature of a room, a thermostat senses the changes and triggers additional functions to keep the room within a range of comfort by turning on a heating or cooling source. Once the ambient temperature returns to that zone, it shuts off. It responds to the room, and the room responds to it, just like people do with one another.

FST is also influenced by several social science theories:

o Structural functionalism mutually prioritizes systemic stability and a desire for homeostasis, or a standard norm. They also both embrace the role of community in developing and maintaining that norm.
o Social exchange and affect theories share an emphasis on the cost/benefit balance in decision-making, assuming people act in the most beneficial and least costly way, taking into account both independent and interdependent (relational) factors.
o Self-regulatory theory looks at what helps people to regulate themselves and set goals, like social standards, motivation to meet those, monitoring threats to the standard, and willpower of the individual. These are enforced by relationships through negotiation, coercion, and induction. These are examples of cybernetics and circular influence.
o The developmental task model looks at forces that alter family adaptability, specifically individual development, shifting systemic roles across life stages, and changes in family structure and situation.

Of course, both humankind and these theories are more complex than these simplified summaries.

FST Core Concepts

While there are numerous theories that contributed to FST, it also has defining features that make it unique from these. CRT pulls from FST's core concepts to understand relationship functionality and opportunities for compassion in systems. The FST concepts are context; co-occurring systems; wholeness; communication, including boundaries; and circular causality. The FST concepts just listed are also present in CRT.

Context

Your context is the physical, social, and emotional settings of our emotional logic – it is why we do what we do. Context is inevitable and ongoing, and it impacts people's authenticity and openness moment-to-moment.

Physical context is your worldly environment, the space you're in and what fills it. These are your immediate settings, often influencing your sensory stimulation: Private versus public spaces; being indoors or outdoors; the presence or absence of natural tones and textures; how crowded a space is or the presence or absence of specific characters in it; climate or temperature; time of day, week, or year; presence of sounds, lights, textures, and so many other factors impacting our physical presence.

Social context is the overt and covert expectations of a person based on socially placed rules and one's roles within those. These can be cultural values, often associated with cultural mores (rules of ethics and morality) and cultural norms (window of expected and accepted behaviors). These rules dictate what are acceptable interactions in different physical settings ("Keep your voice down in a library") or relationships ("Don't talk that way to your mother!").

A person's social roles are the responsibilities you hold in a situation. Roles convey the distribution of power, or hierarchy, in a system. Responsibilities can include behavioral tasks (such as a parent disciplining their child) or emotional tasks (perceived responsibility of a child not to upset their parent). Roles are frequently rooted in relationship with others' roles, such as student and teacher, parent and child, or between two spouses.

Lastly, an additional attribute of social context is distribution of energy. People have to choose on which roles and systems to prioritize their time, effort, resources, and identity, both moment-to-moment and in the long term.

Emotional context is the internal experience of interacting with your physical and social contexts. The internal experience is based on a spectrum of tolerance between comfort and ease to distress and pain. Our past, present, and future contribute to the internal emotional experience of a moment or a memory. Previous experiences with certain people, places, times of year, topics, situations, rules, roles, and responsibilities can convolute current experiences or expectations for the future. Problems can come from how we make sense of those life events (past, present, and future!), and make assumptions rooted in those, such as what we "should" have done or what it says about a person for responding in a way that they later regret. This piece, in particular, is where CRT steps in and approaches counseling differently.

A phrase you will see frequently in this book is that all things make sense in context. When we know more about someone's previous thought process, their emotional wellbeing at the time, and the widespread influencing factors at the moment, we have a better idea why someone says, does, or feels the way they do now or did previously.

Context is also open to fluid interpretation, which means it is changeable. As described in the theory of social constructivism (we'll talk more about this in Chapter 6), your perception, or personal meaning-making, is rooted in your individuality. People can emotionally experience the same space differently, both physically and socially, often based on unique genetic characteristics and meaning-making practices. Therefore, even when individuals grow up or work in the same space, their shared systemic setting does not mean a shared systemic experience.

Co-Occurring Systems

Co-occurring systems is an ecological theory adopted by FST that looks at one's roles in multiple systems, simultaneously. Ecologically, there are five layers of co-occurring systems that can be visualized like a sequence of circles, rippling outward as their influence expands:

- *Immediate self* is the individual person, who can hold multiple perspectives of themselves, attempting to make sense of conflicting messages experienced in life.
- *Microsystems* are one's immediate environment and direct personal relationships.
- *Mesosystems* are where microsystems overlap, such as parental involvement in school events or inviting a colleague from work to a casual event with friends.
- *Exosystems* are the other microsystems of people in your microsystem, such as a romantic partner's workplace or sibling's peer group. Even without direct contact, these systems impact us through our shared person(s).
- *Macrosystems* are one's social and cultural contexts. At this system level, connections are more conceptual (e.g., values, belief systems) than tangible, though occasionally rooted in geographic commonalities, such as individualistic and collectivistic cultures.
- *Chronosystems* are changes and consistencies over short and long spans of time, such as the global context that defines social norms in that era.

Early in life, we define ourselves solely by our systems. As we get older, cognitive development increases self-awareness, and we develop an identity beyond our social contexts, now rooted in one's values, interests, and sense of purpose. However, we also maintain our relational nature with others,

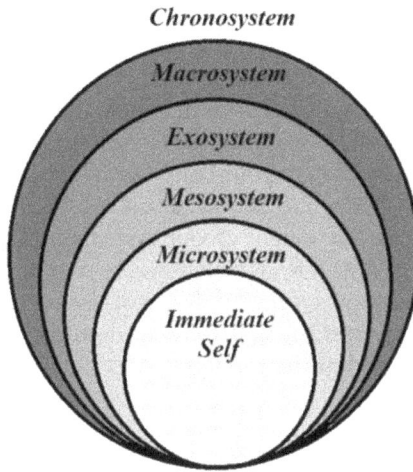

Figure 2.1 Co-Occurring Systems

balancing an identity individually and in communities. In families, early FST theorists simplified these:

- *Suprasystems* are large systems, such as external environments and communities that contribute to a system's identity, values, and beliefs. These include extended families, racial and ethnic subcultures, and religious affiliations, and sports team fan bases.
- *Subsystems* are the smaller divisions and dynamics between members of a system, such as parenting teams or siblings, often in pairs and triads.

A subsystemic structure unique to FST is the relational triangle. Murray Bowen, an early pivotal player in the design of therapeutic application of FST, considers a triad, or triangles, the most stable relational structure. When there is distress in a dyad, a third person may be brought in, theoretically to help stabilize the pair's stress by giving validation, new perspectives, and reminders of skills or alternative courses of action. A therapist, for example! As an added complication, triangles can be interlocking, meaning multiple triangles impact one another.

Unfortunately, when it comes to triangles, some third parties end up destabilizing the pair further when their own biases and desires intervene. Or maybe the third person falls into the role of managing the relationship between the other two people, like a tie-breaker or decision-maker. This is called triangulation. Sometimes in therapy we have heard people use the terms interchangeably. For clarification, *triangles* are the relational structure; *triangulation* can occur between members of the triangle once established! The challenge is to responsibly remain emotionally differentiated enough to be helpful – "stay in your lane," so to speak.

As a final, compassion-based note about co-occurring systems, it is important to recognize the extent of our systems' influence, intentionally and unintentionally. These different systems are part of our social contexts, and as a suprasystem grows larger, it does not negate the intricacies of the subsystems; it incorporates them. Together, these contribute to a person's whole sense of being and of their unique and special role in the systems of which they are a member.

Wholeness

Remember when I said, "The whole is greater than the sum of its parts"? That is what holism is about. Each member of a system is simultaneously part of a larger whole and an independent entity. For example, a geographical territory can be an independent entity and part of a larger system, such as a country or continent. The challenge of any individual, therefore, is finding balance between social integration and autonomy. This is where self-differentiation comes into play. We are constantly trying to find the balance between being part of something else while also recognizing that we are our own person in the midst of that.

Holism looks at each person's creative synthesis. Creative synthesis is the dynamic relationship between a person's past, present, and future (their context!) and how those interact within a person and with other people. The goal is to be whole within ourselves and within our role of a system.

So what are the implications of this perspective? It means the client is not an individual floating in the vacuum of space. They bring with them their context, their roles in their multitudes systems, and their relationships with each of these. The identified patient is, ultimately, the relationships within a person and/or between people. It means an issue in a relationship is never one-sided; if it affects the relationship, it affects all individuals in it.

Communication

So much goes into how people communicate. It falls into two categories: The *digital*, or words, which offer the face-value message, also called the report. The *analog* communication includes the nonverbal cues and conveys the metamessage, or command. Nonverbal cues include tone, volume, body position, and gestures.

FST includes three principles of communication:

1. One cannot not communicate (even silence or turning away communicates a message).
2. One cannot not behave (all behavior is an action, even the action of stillness).
3. Meaning given is not always meaning meant (or meaning intended).

These three principles will be pivotal in circular causality, as discussed later in this chapter.

In addition to these principles, FST highlights three communication styles that impact relationship interactions. Communication styles focus on the nonverbal communication patterns in a relationship:

o Symmetrical, or matching styles
o Complementary, or inverted styles

To figure out which is true for someone, consider this: When someone talks to you loudly and passionately, do you match their energy or respond with a quiet tone (or silence)? If your answer is "it depends," you may qualify for the last style:

o Parallel, which is situationally appropriate symmetry or complementary styles

Communication styles can shift depending on everything from mood to role with the person to setting. (I bet you expect me to say "context" here; that would be correct.)

To send and receive communication includes three levels of interpretation:

Syntactic, or digital interpretation, is the use of the correct words for the intended subject, and whether or not the other person knows those definitions.

Semantic, or interpretation of meaning, is the accurate understanding of how the speaker is using a word, such as words with more than one meaning.

Pragmatic interpretations are the reading of the speaker's behaviors, or nonverbals. People often say that these speak "louder" than the digital message or are viewed as more truthful to the speaker's underlying command message.

Unfortunately, miscommunication also can occur at any of these interpretations.

What causes communication to fail? Simply put, noise. That could be physical noise in a space, such as other conversations, traffic, or static or lag in electronic conversation, or futile attempts to multitask. It can also be emotional, stemmed from beliefs about the speaker, the relationship with them, their message, and/or oneself. The latter also includes one's emotions, such as feeling overwhelmed. These contribute to an inaccurate receival of the message through faulty meaning-making or inferences. To summarize, it's still all about context!

It seems too obvious to say that communication is a central theme in CRT. Interventions frequently focus on how and what is communicated, particularly those rooted in assumptions, or misinterpretations of meaning or patterns. Additionally, therapy is designed to allow nonjudgmental fluidity of perspective by normalizing miscommunication as a human trait. No one can claim to know the objective truth because no one can be purely objective. Lastly, therapy puts to practice the seeking of clarifications and direct communication. Not everyone thinks the same way or has the same meaning-making process. It's ok to overtly ask for clarity! Creating the comfort to do so is part of one's relationship with self, others, and the idea of asking for something so directly.

Boundaries

Boundaries are the rules that organize a system's interactions and convey who is part of a system and what a person's role may be within it. They are the method of communication to create a sense of safety within relationships and within oneself (self-care). They surreptitiously or directly communicate responsibility and authority in a family system. Boundaries are asserted through the flow – or lack of flow – of information between systems or members of a system.

Boundaries can be physical, mental/emotional, and practical:

- *Physical boundaries* protect your personal space, or "bubble," including physical touch. It can also include your sexual limits, such as how and by whom you consent to sexual communication and/or interaction.
- *Mental* and *emotional boundaries* determine how, when, and to what extent you are comfortable expressing thoughts, ideas, and emotions, or receiving those from others, such as receiving advice or being someone a loved one vents to.
- *Practical boundaries* cover the sharing of materials or possessions and the expectation of those being returned/replenished, along with limits or rules around how time is spent, such as how much free time is dedicated to others, setting a realistic schedule for oneself, and prioritization.

Broad examples of boundaries can include limiting the times or spaces in which you interact with a person, such as a certain frequency or duration of time together, only meeting in public spaces or with certain people present, or topics that may be considered off-limits, even temporarily.

The degree to which we are willing to adjust these boundaries is our adaptability. These range from diffused (loosely defined and overly lenient) to rigid and strict. In the middle is a balance of the two, demonstrating a balance of structure and flexibility, equipoised connection and separation with our loved ones. Discovering for yourself what is wanted and needed in your boundaries, and reflecting on why from a stance of seeking understanding, is a necessary part of a relationship, and is a valuable part of the CRT process.

Ideally, boundaries are clear enough to protect one's independent identity within a unifying system but permeable enough to ensure mutual support and sense of comradery. With CRT, the hope is for decreased extremism by not leaping to relational cut-offs, or having permission to change boundaries, such as flexibility based on situation, stage of life, etc.

It is difficult to talk about boundaries without talking about entitlement. When most people think of entitlement, they think of the destructive entitlement, or assumptions of what is inherently due from others. Constructive entitlement, however, is the mutually beneficial balance of fair returns without keeping a ledger. It is an understanding that boundaries are nonthreatening to relationships because there is still a multidirectional balance of influence.

We'll go into boundaries more, including specific steps and skills, in Chapter 9.

Circular Causality

When some people think of a problem, it is human instinct to try and identify the source – Where did it begin? This linear thinking assumes a set start point that triggered the current problem, and if we can find it and shift course, that will presumably fix it. It uses an 'if, then' view of a problem's presence and maintenance. Linear perspective is people who say, "If this one thing was better, everything would be fine!"

Instead, circular causality focuses on the recursive reasons that problems linger; everyone contributes to an ongoing cycle of influence. What you say, do, and feel impacts what others say, do, and feel, which in turn affects how you respond. Any supposed starting point is still influenced by the contexts of what came before it. This cyclical view of interaction helps us understand how someone may be causing their problems to stick around, intentionally or unintentionally.

Cycles of interaction are made of feedback loops. *Positive feedback* encourages the previous behavior. *Negative feedback* discourages it. Positive or negative loops are not titles to indicate they are good or bad. It's akin to reinforcing versus punishing the behavior by encouraging it to continue or not. These tools are frequently used to teach social norms. Either positive or negative feedback have the potential to perpetuate or create constructive or problematic interaction cycles.

We most often see negative feedback loops in situations where someone wants things to stay the way they are. This is called a system's homeostasis, or maintaining of the status quo, such as by negative feedback. This is a natural human desire for predictability, related to the emotional context of comfort. Sociologist Watson Burgess observed that families do not have to be harmonious to be functional, but how we interact is key to both harmony and functionality, both individually and in relationships. Human tendency is to return to patterns and interactions of familiarity, even when dysfunctional.

Another aspect of FST's theory of circularity and change is its inevitability, either through non-purposeful drift or intentionality. Intentional change can come organically, or through normal development; incidentally through atypical life experiences; or intentionally by perturbing the norm. The latter is what happens when a person reaches a point that staying the same is more uncomfortable or painful than the prospect of entering the unknown and abstract "different."

Once change is initiated, it can be in one of two forms. First order is solely behavioral change – the action changes but the mindset stays the same. Research shows these changes are more likely to be temporary because there is less investment from the client to maintain the change. In these cases, the change is typically externally motivated, such as doing something to make someone else happy. When that relationship gets rocky, such as when you get in a fight with that person whose happiness was previously your motive, your motivation to keep the behavior change rocks with it. On the other hand, second order change is a shift in meaning-making cognitively, emotionally, and as a result, behaviorally. This is the function of CRT – to change your emotional relationships with perceived problems in order to approach them differently mentally and behaviorally.

CRT uses FST's theory of change rooted in circularity to acknowledge the craving for comfort as normal. It also recognizes the ease of turning toward the familiar as a way of seeking comfort: "Better the enemy I know than the one I don't." But when we reflect on our past contributions to a problem, there remains space to respond differently without harshness toward our past self because the circular response makes sense in the fullness of our contexts.

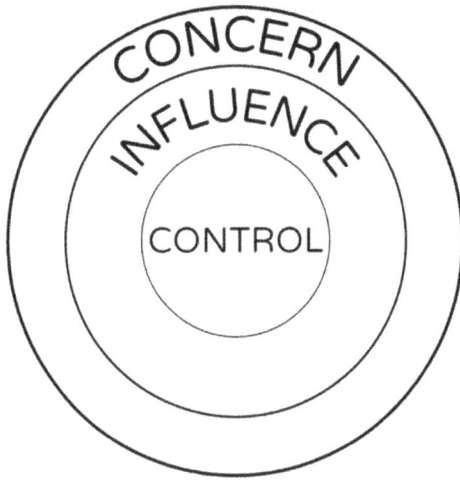

Figure 2.2 Circles of Control, Influence, & Concern

Not only that, but FST shows that one person responding differently can shift the whole system; one positive feedback motion in a cycle begins a deviation in a relationship. If one person changes how they interact with someone else, it can change the relationship itself and the perceptions of the people in it. This is a statement of hope – you really, truly do make a difference all by yourself! Every individual has the potential to influence change in their systems' functioning.

We use the word influence here very intentionally because the use of feedback loops is different from attempts to control. In therapy, we specify that all relationships fall into one of three circles (see Figure 2.2).

These circles, based on Stephen Covey's version in his book *The Seven Habits of Highly Effective People*, portray a division between what a person controls, influences, and what concerns them despite a lack of either control or influence. The innermost circle, the circle of control, is restricted to only what you directly control, such as what you say and do, you attitude or mindset, and your mood or work ethic. You may not necessarily always feel in control of these, such as when we experience automatic thoughts or reactive emotions. The idea of this circle is that you have the capacity to control these, and they are yours to manage and take responsibility for.

The middle circle is more expansive. It encompasses that which we directly influence but do not control. These include others' choices, priorities, actions, thoughts, and emotions, and how they communicate those to you. It also includes how others perceive you; as scary as it seems, those are not fully within your control. Often, I remind clients that the influence circle could sometimes be called the "illusion of control" circle. Because realistically, we can influence others, even heavily influence them, but their choices remain their own. In this way, we can reiterate where responsibilities lie within the perpetuation of problematic interaction cycles.

- Responsibility is taking accountability for your role.
- Blame is the attempt to place responsibility on others.
- Mutual, shared responsibility recognizes not just one person is at fault. It also does not necessarily indicate equal responsibility, though it is not a competition.

The outermost layer is the circle of concern, of no control or influence. These are areas that we do not influence but are influenced by. They just happen, or have already happened, and when they are a focal point in our lives, feelings of helplessness can come too easily. This could be anything from the weather to traffic, to the outcome of a sporting event, to government policy, and the global economy. No wonder it can feel so overwhelming! However, I would say we still have influence over how we experience the circle of concern. I give the metaphor to my clients, you can't change the weather, but you get to decide whether or not to bring an umbrella.

The purpose of these distinctions is to reiterate what is someone's to take ownership over fully (control), versus those that are influential and largely able to be influenced, versus that which can be influential on a macrosystemic level but difficult or impossible to directly influence (concern). Providing psychoeducation about these distinctions will be one of the many responsibilities of the therapist in FST and CRT.

Unique Attributes/Role of the Systemic Therapist

Like CRT, the role of the family systemic therapist is to provide guidance and nonjudgmental curiosity addressing the client's patterns, hopes, strengths, and hindrances. We offer both knowledge and wisdom, insights, and skills. We prioritize physical and emotional safety, an essential component to create change without the shadow of debilitating shame. To achieve this, FST therapists use three specific skills: Multipartiality, a nonpathologizing stance, and shared expertise.

Multipartiality

Multipartiality is the ability to validate all perspectives simultaneously ("I'm on everyone's side") rather than neutrality ("I'm not taking sides"). This enables a therapist to receive multiple points of view with an open mind and view each person uniquely and without assumptions of the therapist's own.

Nonpathologizing

FST explores a diagnosis like a member of the system. It influences the systems and the system influences the diagnosis and its symptomology. It is a part of the feedback loop (but not all of it!), influencing and influenced by others in the system.

Shared Expertise

FST originally used modern interventions that assumed the therapist was the expert in the room and in the setting of treatment goals. Over time, FST shifted to embrace the postmodern worldview that balances the professional expertise of the therapist with the client's expertise in their lives, particularly their experiences and core needs. It is a move toward collaboration over coaching.

Conclusion

When asked to provide a single sentence summary of Compassionate Relational Therapy, I have often said, "It's the integration of family systems theory and compassion-based therapies." Family systems theory, one of the foundational theories contributing to CRT's conceptualizations, is rooted in well-researched and extensive observations regarding human behaviors. The beginning ideas of general systems theory and cybernetics expanded to include social and human tendencies, such as those described by structural functionalism, social exchange theory, social affect theory, self-regulatory theory, and the developmental task model. From there, FST organized its own core principles of interactions and relationships. These are context, co-occurring systems, wholeness, communication and boundaries related to relational hierarchy, and circular causality. When integrated with compassion-oriented practices, we see the impact of and to feedback loops amidst the triadic experience of flowing compassion to self, compassion to others, and compassion from others. Skills specific to systemic therapists that CRT also embraces are multipartiality, nonpathologizing, and shared expertise as we strive to address unwell-ness that is perpetuated by interaction patterns, not just brain chemistry. Between these concepts and those founded on compassion-based thera-pies introduced in Chapter 1, CRT has a foundation from which to build its theory and practices.

Chapter 3

Core Concepts and Skills of Compassionate Relational Therapy (CRT)

Having introduced the contributing founding theories, this chapter explores the core concepts of CRT. We will discuss underlying assumptions; how CRT creates lasting, positive change interpersonally and intrapersonally; and the role of the therapist in CRT. Lastly, we cover the potential and known limits of CRT therapeutically.

Core Concepts of CRT

There are six foundational principles that inform the CRT perspective as clinicians. These premises inform our perceptions about people and the world; they provide the lens through which we view clients and the work that we do. We recognize that every clinician and every therapeutic method has their own assumptions, and that is okay. This section aims to grant a bit more clarity regarding our viewpoints and why we lean into things in the way that we do. Each principle builds on the ones that came before, scaffolding one change to lead to another. These principles can therefore also provide some structure to the therapeutic process, working from one to the next.

1. Human Experience and Existence is a Collection of Relationships

This initial supposition is rooted in philosophy of retrospective determination and reconstruction – we experience the present based on connections to the past, future, and other variables of the present. That is to say, we have a relationship with something based on previous experiences and current expectations. CRT believes people have relationships with their surroundings, other ideas, objects, and situations, and living beings. The relationships we have with these parts of life heavily inform our meaning-making processes and conclusions.

DOI: 10.4324/9781003518730-4

2. *Everything Makes Sense in Context*

If we recognize our existence as innately relational, we embrace the systemic construct that context is everything! Our relationship with our physical and emotional setting is the context. Those relationships are influencing a moment, a decision, a thought, and an emotion. Therefore, there is logic – albeit it, subjective logic – to those moments, decisions, thoughts, and emotions. When we identify that subjective logic, or emotional logic, as befitting to a situation, we cannot call it purely irrational. We understand how we got there, so to speak.

In CRT, this includes the thoughts, behaviors, and emotions that other modalities might call negative or bad. Of course, there are thoughts and emotions that don't feel pleasant, and that does not mean they (or you!) are personally bad or evil. Similarly, there are actions that are undeniably hurtful and problematic. Acknowledging how we got to the point of completing those acts is not the same as condoning or supporting them. There is a significant difference between validation versus agreement. Agreement isn't our goal. For CRT, validation is rooted in understanding the other person's context leading to their outcome, including attributes they could or could not control. This concept sets the foundation for context without judgment or shame. With CRT, we can create a space where clients can look at all aspects of themselves, even emotions like contempt, and integrate understanding with compassion.

3. *Psychoeducation is One Key to Insight through Normalizing and Validation*

Insight toward ourselves increases capacity for self-examination and self-reflection. When we have insight, it increases the tendency to not personalize, isolate, criticize ourselves or those around us. We are able to more objectively view situations, interactions, and emotions. Insight helps us to contextualize and makes it easier to view things in a more objective perspective.

That being said, psychoeducation is more than insight. Psychoeducation is learning about norms and health tied in with the self-compassionate concept of shared humanity and common human experiences. Psychoeducation is the shameless teacher that reiterates you are not alone in your suffering because all people suffer, and all degrees of suffering are hard. It's not a comparison ("Well, they have it worse than me"), nor is there an assumption that having the information will instantly create motivation to change. Research has shown that having insight does not create behavioral change. The purpose of psychoeducation in CRT is to validate and normalize human experiences and challenges without judgment.

4. Self-judgment is the chasm between insight and change

When we feel shame and engage in self-criticism, we call this self-judgment. Self-judgment is labeling and demeaning ourselves, often based on an action (or inaction), thought, or emotion. It is not only the absence of self-kindness; it is the overt presence of personalization and felt isolation. Self-judgment perpetuates harshness toward oneself. Even when we know better (insight), that is used against us instead of to motivate us to make change. CRT believes this is the gap that stops change from happening: self-judgment and shame.

Another way to put this is that self-judgment is where we notice people get "stuck" in therapy. Other modalities may even call this "resistance." In CRT, we view this as an absence of or hesitance toward compassionate practices, interventions, or language. Clients can experience resistance to compassion for a few different reasons, such as apprehension toward compassion's meaning, process, or applicability/trust in its usefulness to solve their current problems. For example, if someone believes that having compassion equates to a lack of accountability, or that compassion for themselves feels entirely foreign, then they might be more hesitant to try. Right away, we want to acknowledge that this isn't a bad thing; there isn't shame around this hesitance. We recognize there is context to it, even if that context is misinformation. Either way, it begins with discomfort, and we can be compassionate toward that feeling. Everyone starts in a different space when it comes to their compassion journey. In CRT, we hope that through time, safety, exploration, and preparedness, clients can begin to examine themselves and those compassion blocks with the greater objectivity that comes with nonjudgmental curiosity, paving the way forward for compassion to grow.

5. Crossing the chasm of self-judgment requires compassion via nonjudgmental curiosity

Nonjudgmental curiosity is when we compassionately engage in questions about someone's life or experience without expectations or assumptions. In order to experience authentic compassion for self and others, we need to hold that there is not one right way to think, feel, or act. Nonjudgmental curiosity allows us to ask questions and gather context, seeking to understand more in order to better empathize. The more context we have, the better, especially when it comes to developing empathy and compassion. It also gives us the opportunity to differentiate excuses from explanations, looking at where someone can take accountability for their contributions to context, too. At this point in therapy, we hope to help clients prioritize listening to understand, not judge or correct the other person. Oftentimes, a lack of awareness or acknowledgement makes it harder to lean into understanding or acceptance. People are better listeners when they feel heard; we make sure they first feel heard and validated by us, the therapist, to help them regulate their emotions and stay in the present. Once able to do this, we help our clients grow in their listening and validating toward one another and themselves. Nonjudgmental curiosity also allows the therapist to explore circularity in the relationship, such as asking nonjudgmentally how one person would guess the other is feeling in a moment.

6. Compassion is both an emotional disposition and learnable skill

Integrating all the above foundational beliefs, CRT poses that compassion is both an emotional disposition and a skill we can learn and integrate into our lives and relationships. Mindfulness and kindness are both states of being and skills. Awareness of our shared human suffering without comparison may require intentionality to reiterate to oneself. Compassion, like any form of growth, takes time and care. People do not suddenly shift from self-critical to self-compassionate; if the transition were that linear, we would all have done it already. Instead, every instance of self-criticism is a new opportunity for self-compassion.

Compassion is an act of intimacy. This is a method for second order change; we are not just changing behavior but changing the underlying foundation of how someone presents themself and how they interact with the world. Depending on how clients integrate and use compassion for self and others, how they lean into assumptions about self or other changes as well. If we believe that we are worthy and deserving of kindness, gentleness, softness, and grace, how we approach ourselves and situations will look different. Our goal is effort, not a singular outcome. We can finetune, adjust and workshop communication once we have the foundation of compassionate relational safety. Healing happens in the observed and validated effort to do and think differently and love graciously and authentically. That is where compassion grows.

How CRT Creates Change

CRT believes that change is created through learning to utilize the skill or compassion, grow the skill, and increase understanding and accessibility of skill. Once you learn compassion for self and others, the ability to do so never goes away. It's like riding a bike.

Of course, CRT isn't the only therapy modality that believes that learning and using new skills creates change. There are aspects of CRT that draw from other therapeutic modalities such as Emotion-Focused Therapy,

Narrative Therapy, Internal Family Systems, and Gottman's Couples Therapy. While this is not an attachment-based model we acknowledge the strengths of attachment-based models and their empirical validity. Where we differ is that in CRT, the focus is not overtly to create secure attachment in external relationships. If anything, it is to create secure attachment within oneself through self-compassion, which research has shown improves capacity for compassion toward others. The difference is not only the interventions but the specific and intentional focus on increasing self-kindness and decreasing judgment toward self and others as a means to improve personal and relational resilience. This resilience is the ability to connect and communicate with yourself and others in a healthier and more authentic way. We invite our clients to share and accept their own experiences and identities, moving toward authentic acceptance of their own selves in order to be able to receive the experiences and identities of their loved ones.

Remember, per the underlying theory of CRT, people exist in a collection of relationships. Those relationships may be temporary, long term, deep, shallow, passive, active, etc. In the context of therapy, both the therapist and client are actively engaging with one another and the perceived problem and the emotional experiences that accompany it. CRT emphasizes that we have a relationship with our problems separate from ourselves and our loved ones. We are seeking to improve the relationship with the problem by offering it compassion, recognizing how it has not always been a problem, and reflecting on what a solution can look like with it.

Our theory of change has three main points to it. We believe that if these three components can be actively and fluidly present in our clients' lives and relationships, then growth, learning, and compassion will be more present:

1. When we feel heard and understood, we are more resilient, receptive to change, and more compassionate to self and others.
2. Healing comes from the effort, not the outcome, of therapy.
3. When we approach people with nonjudgmental curiosity, we minimize the perpetuation of shame and the resulting "stuckness" that can often come from that.

All those points touch on the core concepts of CRT: authentically hearing perspectives of others, receiving compassion from others, putting in effort toward the healing, and non-judgment from therapist and partners.

Role of the CRT Therapist

Research about therapeutic effectiveness has consistently shown the therapeutic relationship between the provider and client is a leading contributor to positive therapeutic outcomes. Therefore, the role of the CRT therapist is, primarily, to intentionally foster that relationship through demonstration of nonjudgmental curiosity and providing examples of compassion-driven language for the client. As a CRT therapist, we exemplify and embody compassion for self and others actively in session.

Factors that contribute to the compassionate therapeutic relationship and, as a result, therapeutic outcomes, include therapist multipartiality, warmth and friendliness, and the ability to listen attentively. In practice, this can look very similar to person-centered, or Rogerian, therapy. This prioritizes psychological safety through nonjudgment, congruence, and supportive presence, trademarked as unconditional positive regard for the client. CRT maintains that philosophy and utilizes the model's two major interventions to achieve this – active listening and reflection:

- *Active listening* is conveyed through attentive body posture and nonverbal cues (nodding, appropriate facial expressions and utterances, etc.).
- *Reflection* is two-fold. It includes both the summarization of what is said, or the content of the client's statements (including use of the client's language). It is also noticing aloud the perceived emotional experience of the client both in the present moment ("Thank you for sharing that; I imagine that was very difficult to tell me") or about the material shared ("I could see that situation having been very anxiety-inducing; was that your experience, or did you feel something else?").

Active listening and reflecting are innately compassionate qualities therapists can bring to session, both in feedback to and from clients and demonstrated to them to potentially offer others (including one another in multi-person client systems).

While the clients are the experts in their own lives, the therapist brings the psychoeducation, compassion-building skillset, and their own personhood. As a CRT therapist we exemplify and embody compassion for self and others actively in session. We aim to be open, warm, and encouraging. We are also authentic, offering a sense of shared humanity by bringing our own imperfections and "humanness," engaging with clients in a personable way. This self-disclosure is, of course, done professionally and appropriately, with the emphasis consistently on how the client benefits from the sharing. Primarily, we bring the humanness of our own emotions, acknowledging them as they occur in session, and demonstrating how to not villainize or minimize them in the process. The therapist's ability to demonstrate these skills can provide clients with examples of the language they may offer themselves kindly.

A Note from Emma: Oftentimes in my sex therapy work with couples, one of the most reassuring and normalizing things I've said is "you're not the only people in this space who are struggling with this." Clients want to know that their therapist understands how tricky life can be. It can be additionally challenging to show up to therapy and have a therapist who seems "perfect," "faultless," and free of human struggle. It can be very isolating for clients to feel like they are the only people experiencing certain challenges, and CRT wants to decrease that sense of alienation and isolation. Knowing the therapist is a human who also experiences hardship can be very comforting and rapport building.

Research in the past decade endorses that therapist mindfulness contributes to perceived alliance and leads to an increased passion for the clinical work. Additionally, self-compassion poses numerous benefits to the clinician:

- Enhance empathic accuracy
- Moderate unpleasant emotions (worry, rumination, self-criticism) after ambivalent feedback
- Increase individuals' self-reflection and acknowledgement of their role in negative events without feeling overwhelmed
- Improve alliance and perceived approachability
- Improve cognitive flexibility
- Decrease people-pleasing tendencies (including toward the client)

All this leans into therapist authenticity, a significant factor in therapist perceived trustworthiness. To achieve the desired dynamic and avoid transference problems, it is essential the therapist be authentically present with clients rather than having an emotionally distanced professional demeanor. The therapist must be willing to do their own self-of-the-therapist work. These can include building one's own genogram; interviewing one's family of origin to learn family strengths and legacies; creating a personal timeline of significant events personally, in the family, communally, and culturally; previously identified experiential exercises; story-telling groups of therapists; or groups of therapists doing self-of-the-therapist work together, witnessing to one another. The goal is to experience and provide an environment where it is safe to identify various contexts and perspectives. The creation of this safety starts with therapists modeling this compassion. They also fold well into allyship with and for the client.

CRT Therapist as Ally

It is also important to recognize that CRT therapists lean in toward ally-ship, shared accountability/"imperfect solidarity" to counter problematic narratives, including microaggressions. Here are some core aspects of being an ally in CRT:

1. There isn't one right and singular way to be an ally – what matters most is the belief you have for your clients in who they are and how they identify.
2. Our goal is to create a space where clients can safely exist as their authentic selves.
3. We invite clients to identify any inadvertent microaggression they experience from us without fear of negative consequence (non-judgment!).
4. We want clients to experience the safety of expressing their needs.
5. Being an ally isn't only identified by attending public events or publicly posting. This can also be identified through the language we use and the ways we interact.

Potential Limits of CRT

While we do believe in the strengths of CRT, we would be remiss if we didn't mention the dynamics where CRT may not be as beneficial. Therefore, there are a few limitations of CRT: psychosis, limited cognitive development, discernment counseling, or the presence of relational therapy contraindicators (the "3 A's").

Psychosis

We fully recognize that this modality requires an ability to think constructively, clearly, and introspectively about self and others. When people experience psychosis, such as in schizophrenia, the brain has less cognitive flexibility and poor memory. Compassion-building may be challenged by loose relationship with reality or delusion-based assumptions. That being said, psychosis does not make CRT impossible; more likely there will be individual compassion work first to learn how to talk about it without being ruled by stigmatization. Delusional symptoms could be viewed as personal or relational narratives to disentangle, and parts language has been shown to help people contextualize hallucinations and intrusive thoughts. However, overall, psychosis could make engaging with interventions more challenging, such as exploring underlying emotions contributing to relationship dynamics and navigating clear and constructive thoughts and plans.

Limited Cognitive Development

Compassion requires us to reflect beyond concrete thought and deal with metacommunication. Certain developmental thinking processes and capabilities don't solidify until individuals reach the formal operations stage of cognitive development. While this often occurs at a certain age for people, that is not always the case. Therefore, younger children or adults who aren't at this stage of development could find it harder to benefit from CRT.

Discernment Counseling

Distinct from couples' therapy, discernment counseling hopes to determine whether the pair want to stay together or not. If a couple doesn't want to understand one another's perspective or cultivate compassionate safety to be authentic in one's needs, CRT will not be as applicable. However, if they are in discernment counseling because they want to use nonjudgmental curiosity toward one another and their potential future options, CRT individual therapy could be a fit. People can have relationships with and meaning-making about ideas such as divorce or separation that could be addressed. Because we are so focused on the relational aspect, there is a baseline level of commitment to interpersonal work necessary to get the most out of CRT.

Contraindications for Relational Therapy

When working with relationships, such as families and romantic relationships, another limit of CRT would be if there is active presence of the common contraindicators in the presenting relationship. These are often referred to as the "3 A's": addiction/substance abuse, current physical or sexual abuse, and affairs. When immediate danger is a variable, CRT wouldn't be conducive, since the priority in these situations is to resolve the danger at hand. If the therapeutic space does not feel safe to be authentic, compassion will be at a standstill. Before we can grow compassion, there has to be a baseline level of safety and interpersonal functioning. In the case of current addiction and abuse, working toward recovery and symptom- and risk-management are the first priorities.

In many people's lives, there can be past addiction or abuse (in the current relationship or in previous relationships) and ongoing emotional, mental, or verbal abuse. We know life and relationships are complicated and can be messy. We want CRT to be available to those who have encountered all types of life experience. If physical abuse was a previous part of the current relationship, we would work with the individuals to identify the context of the abuse and create a plan for what we would do if abuse resurfaces. We would also want to ensure that additional support, such as group therapy, individual therapy, and/or peer or medical support were part of the holistic care the clients receive. Similarly with affairs and addictions, if this was a part of a past relationship or previous season in life, we view these as context to the current story and have open conversation about each person's relationship with those memories. In CRT, if we see that substance use, affairs, and/or abuse surface during therapy, treatment would redirect to management, support, safety establishment, and termination if necessary.

Conclusion

CRT works from the core belief that we exist in relationship to the world around us, building meaning-making on experiences of the past and present and ideations about the future. These are our context, and our context always makes sense and offers subjective logic to why we act, think, and feel the ways we do in any given moment. With a combination of this reflection and psychoeducation pertaining to social norms and wellbeing, we can validate ourselves and others without judgment, shame, or criticism. When we are able to do this, a bridge appears spanning the chasm between insight and change. That bridge is compassion between ourselves and others, both giving and receiving. CRT aims to create compassion in people both as an emotional temperament and skill. Compassion works to nurture resilience through both kindness and accountability, which is how the change occurs. CRT therapists oversee this process as a guide, providing direction while also demonstrating the skills themselves. While CRT is designed to reach the widest audience, there are limitations. That being said, the process of CRT treatment, from intake through discharge, aims to encourage emotional fortitude through softness, not callousness.

Chapter 4

CRT Stages of Therapy

One of the most valuable parts of therapy modalities is the techniques they use to create and maintain change. CRT has a flexible structure without set timelines. The therapy process can be brief or prolonged; treatment can take the time needed for lasting change and growth.

In this chapter, we cover CRT intake material and approach to assessment. We then identify interventions of CRT, which can occur across all stages of therapy, including assessment. Lastly, we look at the recommended processes for the closure of treatment when the time comes.

In CRT, there is not a designated order for intake and assessment questions, nor an order for the interventions to be utilized. You may notice assessment and intervention even intermingle as we constantly learn more about our clients throughout the therapy process. In this chapter, we offer possible phrasing for questions; these are not scripts. Since authenticity is an essential therapeutic quality in CRT, it is important for clinicians to phrase questions in terms that feel most natural to them and compatible with the clients.

Intake Material

The intake is a space for therapist and client to become more acquainted with one another and identify hopes for the therapeutic outcome. The therapist will offer a groundwork of compassionate language from this very first session. The intake serves purposes:

- Provide an overview of the therapy process
- Initial sense for clients' current capacity to give/receive compassion for self and others
- Assess for therapeutic contraindications

DOI: 10.4324/9781003518730-5

Providing an Overview of Therapy

In CRT intakes, we immediately work to create a space of safety by overtly providing an overview of the therapy process, identifying what to expect. This would cover:

1. Introduction of the therapist and relevant credentials
2. Summary of the systemic and compassion-rooted therapeutic philosophy for meaningful and lasting change
3. What to expect therapy to include, such as emotional and behavioral potential benefits and challenges
4. Structure of therapy, such as periodic individual or dyadic sessions as part of relational therapy
5. Review of informed consent, confidentiality limits, and secret-keeping policies

An example of setting expectations can include expectations of attendance, including who attends, frequency of sessions, and timeliness. When working with a relationship, at least half of the sessions will be as the relationship unit. Ideally, the first session will be together with subsequent individual sessions. In the breakout sessions, therapists can assess for past and current individual and relational trauma and re-affirm the absence of contraindications.

After the initial joint and individual sessions, the clients and therapist collaborate to decide how often they want to meet as a system versus individually. For example, they may prefer two sessions together followed by individual sessions, or they can do more consistent sessions together with fewer individual sessions interspersed. CRT balances relational and individual sessions to provide holistic care to the client system. Individual sessions can offer opportunity for the clients to dive deeper into their selves, discern what contributes to their sense of safety and security, and identify possible blocks for compassion when they may not yet feel ready to share these with loved ones.

Any time therapists work with multiple members in a client system, it is important to identify your secret-keeping policy. Because the clients' relationship is viewed as the therapeutic client, content in individual sessions is considered appropriate to include in together sessions. We may not be the first to bring the material up, but we may ask, *"What would it be like to talk to your loved one about this?"* It is not helpful to the therapeutic relationship for the therapist to be a secret-keeper or "tattler" for either member of the client system.

Initial Capacity for Compassion

Inevitably, clients begin therapy wanting to talk about what brings them in at this time in their lives. How they talk about those experiences, those memories, and the people involved in them (including themselves) will begin to indicate their level of compassion or capacity to value and see multiple perspectives. While talking through this, the therapist will also begin to validate them, potentially both their actions *("That makes sense!")* and their thoughts or feelings *("I could understand that")*. Here is where we notice how receptive they are to this, too. Are they critical of themselves and push off the validation? Are they eager for it? Do they weaponize it toward anyone else in the room? These are all part of this intake and the start of therapeutic assessment.

Understanding the baseline of each individual's receptivity to compassion will inform the therapist of the treatment starting line and how best to approach and guide the clients.

Assessing for Therapeutic Contraindications

Per standard relational therapy practices, CRT assesses for the contraindications to relationship therapy that were identified in the previous chapter. These would inhibit healing and compassionate connection (addiction, abuse, and affairs). While current physical or sexual abuse are immediate contraindicators, further questioning will be needed if emotional or mental abuse are present. If physical or sexual abuse has previously been part of the relationship, the assessment will also include safety planning as needed. The therapists will need to clarify this language will need to stop in order to build the emotional safety both in the therapy space and outside it. If emotional or mental abuse is present, this will be the first focus in treatment. Here are a few examples of how to ask about that, potentially individually rather than together:

- *"Sometimes in relationships we find ourselves experiencing things we didn't imagine such as addiction, abuse, or affairs. These can often be really hard to talk about, and in this space we want to make sure that all types of conversations can be had. Since we care about you as individuals/together, we want to check in and see if these are things we're experiencing in the relationship. With absolutely no judgment and only compassionate curiosity, are any of these part of what we're experiencing in the relationship?"*
- *"Sometimes we experience things in life that make healing feel more challenging for us. Does it feel for you/either of you like we're experiencing these or that they might be impacting our healing process?"*

Assessment Process and Essential Questions

Initial assessment is typically viewed as the gathering of background and current information that lead up to the initiation for therapy at this time. This can include general informational context such as the presenting problem that lead to starting therapy at this time, living arrangements, known medical and psychiatric stressors, recent solution attempts and contributions to safety, etc. In addition to these, let's explore the components of CRT's assessment process, what we try to look for and understand before diving deeper with our clients. While assessment begins in the first few sessions, it will go beyond the beginning of treatment as we continue to learn and evaluate with our clients throughout the therapeutic process. Even in the early assessment process, compassion is the name of the game. As a generalization, our assessment process will explore:

- Client buy-in regarding the role of compassion in lasting and relational change
- Client self-perception/introspection
- Learning client treatment goals
- Expectations of therapeutic pace

Client Buy-In Regarding the Role of Compassion in Lasting and Relational Change

With every therapy modality, it's important that clients want to do the work. The work of CRT includes establishing validation and compassion as prerequisites/means for change. Since compassion is the basis of CRT, it is important clients believe in the power of compassion and have desire to learn about and explore it. To assess this, the therapist might ask, "*What do you think of when I say words like validation and compassion?*" Listen for if they are dismissive or minimizing, or eager to agree. Do they correctly understand the concepts, or do they have misconceptions about either? If clients are hesitant about compassion, the therapist may ask, "*What do you believe might happen if you give yourself or your loved one compassion?*" Psychoeducation may be needed. This can also be an overall assessment for readiness to change.

At this stage, we are also listening for the use of feelings language overall. We want to see how or if the clients access and identify their emotions and conceptualize them. We also want to see if it seems hard for them to access their emotions, voice that which they're feeling, or even find value in doing so. A way to check on this may be to ask, "*How do you feel about starting this counseling process?*" or, "*How does it feel to hear me validate that/you?*" Wherever they are in in their emotional attunement, there's no shame or judgment; it's helpful for us to know so we can adjust which skills we focus on first.

Client Self-Perception/Introspection

How our clients talk about themselves can be a huge indicator of their self-perception, introspection, and self-compassion. How they describe themselves, their experiences, and others can provide valuable insight to their degree of self-kindness, mindfulness, and sense of shared humanity versus self-criticism, personalization, and isolation.

- Do clients use harsh and degrading language to describe themselves and situations? (Example client statement: "I shouldn't be like this, I need to get over how my partner hurt me, I can't believe that I'm so stupid and stuck," versus, "This isn't my favorite part about myself, but I recognize this is where I'm growing. What my partner did was hurtful, and it's taking me time to get through it.")
- Does the client personalize mistakes or failures, or can they offer grace and release after challenges? (Example client statement: "I'm such a failure, I can't believe I messed that up," versus, "I handled this poorly. I can learn from it and do differently in the future.")
- Can clients acknowledge the impact of their words and actions on others? (Example client statement: "They get offended too easily. I can't believe that bothers them," versus, "I can see how that would feel hurtful to them. I'm glad they brought it to my attention.")
- Are their goals for therapy phrased as changes in the relationship or changes in the other person? (Example client statement: "I'm just here to support them, we're here because of them anyway" versus, "We're in this together, and I want to grow too.")

For a quantitative assessment of self-perception, the Self-Compassion Scale (SCS) can supplement this information.

Learn Client Treatment Goals

In CRT, the goals set in therapy should be framed around the self and the relationship, not changes in the other person. If the clients phrase the goals otherwise, the therapist may reflect the stated goal back in a way that is consistent with this structure, or request the client reframe it. It can also help for the therapist to highlight the overlap between the individuals' stated goals. Lastly, therapists phrase goals back to clients in compassion-rooted language. For example, the client might say, "I'm the worst at getting our teen to clean their room, I know it pisses my spouse off." The therapist may reframe this, "It sounds like you recognize that this is not a strong skill of yours, and you want to work on that. What a testament to you and your relationship with both your son and spouse that you see their possible feelings, where growth can happen, and you want to create healthier interactions."

Set Expectation for Pace of Treatment

Everyone arrives at therapy in different headspaces; that is normal. The pace and duration of treatment will vary based on the clients' initial understanding of and openness to applying compassion-rooted practices, gauging client receptivity. The assessment content will inform the therapist where to begin, including setting expectations of the therapy process, and kinds of change it can achieve. A way to describe this could be, *"Compassion for self and others is a muscle in your body; different people tend to use muscles in their bodies uniquely. Your compassion muscles will take time to flex and strengthen. Part of this process is learning what it looks like and how you and your loved ones to use those parts of your body."*

Therapeutic Interventions Consistent with Other Therapies

Built into assessment and expanding beyond it, therapeutic interventions are often viewed as the source of change in therapy. CRT isn't trying to reinvent the wheel, nor are we merely repackaging existing legitimate material into something new. CRT poses a different theory of change than other models: the cultivation of compassion for self and other creates transformative relational and personal healing. This opens new possible applications of known and empirically validated interventions that were introduced in other models of psychotherapy. Here, we identify interventions in CRT made popular by other therapies. In the next chapter, we will introduce the interventions special or unique to CRT.

Keys from Cognitive-Behavioral Therapy (CBT)

As an insurance company favorite, we would be doing a disservice to our readers not to acknowledge a few shared interventions between CRT and CBT. The most substantial is the shared love of psychoeducation – providing new knowledge for insight as a factor to change behavior. We also utilize reframing, which is the intentional shift in language to aid a shift in perspective and exploration of alternative perspectives. Questions such as, *"What else could be true?"* can be very important in both individual and relationship work!

Keys from Compassion-Focused Therapy

As mentioned in the first chapter, CFT paved the way for integrating mindfulness skills in therapy: grounding to the present through our senses; self-soothing for emotional regulation; use of friend-like language; and finding and using compassionate mantras. CRT similarly focuses on compassion flowing out, finding and re-experiencing the emotional and physical sensation of previously experienced compassion. Like CFT's friend-like language, CRT preaches the importance of being the friend, cheerleader, or support figure you need now or needed in the past. In session, therapists may invite clients to reference back to helpful statements and acts by others who care about us and practice offering those to ourselves: *"When you imagine talking to your sister about this, what would you hope she would say?"*

Keys from Emotion-Focused Therapy (EFT)

Despite theoretical differences, the gentle and kind approach of EFT can be applicable in CRT. While not overtly an attachment-based therapy, CRT may use information about attachment styles in psychoeducation and, as said in the previous chapter, prioritizes the therapeutic relationship as a mechanism for change. CRT also uses emotion conjecture, postulating and heightening the possible emotions present to experientially offer compassion in real time. Finally, common to many systemic therapy models, CRT and EFT both lean into intentionally slowing down the session process and material. A therapist may need to jump in on a client's monologue and state, *"Hold on, I'd like us to slow down for a moment and give due acknowledgement to all that was just shared,"* or something similar to interject into a potential slew of new content that could hijack important moments of progress in session if overlooked.

Keys from Solution-Focused Therapy

Solution-focused therapy is famous for its question structures that emphasize progress toward preferred outcomes rather than the problem itself. We have adopted some of these in similar interest to strengths and fostering space for humanness:

- Desired outcome questions (shift verbiage to focus on what we wish was present rather than absent)
- Exception-seeking, coping, and reframing questions (identify occasions when the client overcame a similar issue in the past or could view the problem in a different way)

Throughout treatment, we spotlight client strengths and perseverance through hardships of their lives, including now. Highlighting strengths is an essential compassionate skill to contradict the often-too-quick internal voice of self-criticism/self-judgment. Solution-focused questions normalize the human experiences of emotional ups and downs normalizing emotional ranges and events as part of life.

Metaphors

Clients frequently speak, almost automatically, in metaphors. They use language of "pick your battles," "running on empty," and "needing the right tools." This stems from the basic human skill of storytelling for relatability. CRT welcomes this language, often as part of using the client's language. Clients' metaphors can be carried throughout therapy and indication of progress (*"What does running on half tank look like compared to empty for you?"*). Additionally, we can tweak the metaphor when they are counterproductive. "Pick your battles," for example, assumes the other person is an opponent. Instead, we can say, "Pick your priorities," to reiterate the other person is a teammate, not the competition. "Teammate" becomes the new metaphor we can come back to.

> **A Note from Bethany:** Here's a metaphor I frequently use with clients about the difference between dependence and interdependence in relationships: *"When I am sick with the flu, I am pitiful. I sniffle and stay in bed as much as possible. In those times, when I'm hungry, I can make my own soup. It will be from a can, and I'll lean over the stove to inhale the steam to clear my sinuses, but I can make my own soup. That being said, there is something different about when my partner makes it for me. It might still be from a can, or it might be homemade; either way, it's special when they bring it to me to sip in bed. I can make my own soup, but there's something about my partner doing it for me, both of us knowing I'll do the same for them when they're sick, that makes that soup taste that much better."*

Keys from Satir's Experiential Therapy

Like metaphors, clients often innately use parts language about themselves: "It's like a part of me just didn't want to," or, "A part of me will always love them." CRT embraces this language because it is another way that people make sense of themselves, finding a way for multiple perspectives to coexist within them at the same time, even when they seem to contradict one another. Virginia Satir, an originator of using FST in therapy, utilized this, and demonstrates how we can normalize this and respond to it.

CRT will incorporate conversations about parts of who we are while focusing on compassionately understanding them or coming up with names and titles for them. The clinician can demonstrate the language of what compassionate responses the client needed at different times in their life, then practicing experientially for them to offer that to themselves, such as with a hand over their heart. This can be completed both individually and with client system members present, such as a partner or family member. The goal of this is to emphasize that we do not have to wait to receive these compassionate statements from our loved ones; we are capable ourselves.

Compassionate Relational Interventions

We will go into detail regarding the CRT-specific interventions in the next chapter. For now, we will simply identify them by their categorizations:

- Intentional language, which includes replacing "but" with "and," answering the hypothetical "why," and the use of metaphors and parts language
- Compassionate contextualization
- Disentangling
- Positive restorations, including peaceful pauses, personal and relational check-ins, relationship check-ins, and conversational pauses
- Temporary agreements

A Note from Bethany and Emma: In our first few drafts of this text, the chapters covering the CRT stages of therapy and the CRT interventions formed one giant chapter. It was so long, that on reflection, we decided it might be a lot for readers. We hope this teaser is a fair taste test of what's to come!

Conclusion of Treatment

Ideally, therapy is concluded when the client's goals are completed and compassion is used as a reliable tool for the client, personally and relationally. Refer back to the early intake sessions; we asked how they hope therapy will help them and their relationship, including behavioral and mental changes they would see in themselves and notice in others. The therapist will also consistently look at the clients' interactions with self and others that demonstrates more consistent compassion and ability to receive compassion from others.

How Does the Therapist Convey the End of the Therapy Relationship?

When the therapist notices the predominant presence and receptivity of compassion, it may be up to them to suggest the possibility of concluding treatment. In that conversation the therapist will celebrate the clients' strengths and presence of meaningful change. When doing so, the therapist places emphasis on the clients' contributions to these, not medication, the therapist, or other extra-therapeutic factors. Of course these influence the outcome, but that's not what we're celebrating.

In session, the therapist and client(s) can review goals, reassessing the client's perception of how they are doing on each one. We listen for how they talk about those goals and their role in the changes that have happened. Like with the assessment and intake, the therapist listens for language of compassion for their humanness – past, present, and future. We can also offer opportunities for them to add new goals; if they do so, therapy may continue.

What About When the Client Thinks They're Done, But the Therapist Thinks There's Still Work to Do?

In situations when clients are ready to conclude, we still offer celebration of perceived progress! Their perception is real and full of hope if this is how they feel. From there, we can offer "stepdown" options, if feasible, at your practice site. These could move from weekly to EOW to monthly to as needed, then we would close their file if, after a month, they decide they're emotionally secure to pause therapy, even indefinitely. Sometimes a "stepdown" is not an option, such as when a client needs to end treatment for extra-therapeutic reasons or simply ghosts the therapeutic process. In those cases, it is fair to still celebrate progress, then shift to normalize a future return to treatment, with the same therapist or someone different.

Normalizing a Future Return to Treatment

Therapy is like when you are in a car, and the "check engine" light comes on. Ideally, you will be able to pull over, and a mechanic can come and provide the needed part/tool, maybe even show you how to fix the problem independently in the future. You can get back in the car and keep driving, and the light may come back on. It might be the same issue or a different one, and it might be helpful to reach back out to that mechanic. That's totally understandable; there is always more to learn, in so many parts of life. The therapist may ask, *"How would you know it was time to go back to therapy? How would your life be different then?"* We can encourage the client to write these down for their own reminder, and practice a final compassion statement reiterating this to be a normal part of life and the ongoing relationship with therapy as a helpful option in healing.

Conclusion

CRT uses the three-stage system of psychotherapy including assessment, intervention, and conclusion. In addition to information-based assessment questions, CRT intentionally asks and considers the clients' perceptions of self, others, and compassion as a concept moving into meaningful and lasting change. While integrating some interventions of other therapy models, there are also five key interventions unique to the model, which will be articulated in the next chapter.

Chapter 5

CRT Interventions

In the previous chapter, we identify therapeutic interventions from other therapy models that CRT also utilizes. This chapter is dedicated to interventions that are newly minted to tie with CRT's philosophy of how lasting change happens: once rooted in the safety of internal and interpersonal compassion, people are more able to build personal resilience and accept influence without blame, moving toward prosperous relationships with self and others. To do this, we believe in five essential practices:

- Intentional Language
- Compassionate Contextualization
- Disentangling
- Positive Restorations
- Temporary Agreements

These do not all need to be completed, or completed in a specific order, nor do they have time limits. Many will be used concurrently, like psychoeducation throughout.

Intentional Language

Psychologist and psycholinguist Steven Pinker said, "The language we use influences the way we think." Similarly, famed author, speaker, and social worker Brene Brown has said of language, "Language shows us that naming an experience doesn't give the experience power, it gives us the power of understanding and meaning." A person's language – the words they use both inside their head and out loud – is a reflection of their personal upbringing, larger cultural influence, and social settings. We use the language we hear throughout our lives. Sometimes this is for the better, inspiring hope, resilience, and creativity; sometimes it hinders us into dark patterns of thought and beliefs. It also proves to be a powerful tool in therapy through reframing, as mentioned above. In CRT, there are specific

DOI: 10.4324/9781003518730-6

linguistic interjections we hope to intercede to aid clients in shifting their perspective, including more compassion toward self and others.

Replacing "But" with "And"

Have you ever noticed when someone says something that sounds nice, and then they follow it up with, "*but* . . .," it instantly seems to erase whatever nice thing came before it? The kind statement in the first half of the communication seems to lose its sincerity because the second half overshadows it. This can be especially disheartening when the second half of the message seems contradictory to the first half. Here are some examples:

"I love you, but it drives me crazy when you do that."
"I appreciate what you did, but you should have done it differently."
"I'm sorry you feel that way, but it's not my fault you didn't understand me."

Don't get me wrong, those sentences have a lot more going on than just the *but* in the middle. That being said, see how different even one of these emotion-laden sentences seems with one small change: "I love you, and . . ."

By changing that one word, we have shifted the language to allow that first half of the sentence to coexist with the second half. They no longer erase one another. They also introduce compassionate perspectives that invite further language changes:

"I love you and I have a hard time when you do that."
"I appreciate what you did, and there are other ways to do it, too."
"I wish you didn't feel that way, and I can see how you heard what I said the way you did, even when that wasn't my intention."

A few of these demonstrate the linguistic change of replacing pseudo-sorrys with I-statements reflecting the speaker's feelings and experience through "I wish."

Another example of *and* allows the coexistence of seemingly inconsistent truths about ourselves. In session, the therapist might ask the client, *"What are two things about yourself that are both true despite seeming contradictions within or between them?"* If easier, they may give impersonal reflections, or identify a celebrity or entertainment media (book, movie, etc.) that has parts they both like and dislike.

The purpose of this shift is to reiterate the possibility of loving and accepting someone – including ourselves – amidst imperfections. For ourselves, this could be a question such as, "What was something that you've done that was both hard and good?" With a loved one, it could be, "What is something you love about this person, regardless of the presence of challenging attributes?" Additionally, this creates space for communication's intent *and* impact, not one or the other. This principle also applies to other word alternatives, seeking to replace inflexible (like *always* or *never*) or conditional (*either/or*) language. Doing so brings the reality of the conversation to the forefront where hyperbolic language can feel aggressive or insurmountable.

Answering the Hypothetical "Why"

Have you ever noticed that when someone asks you why you do something, a little defensiveness almost automatically pops up in you? Or maybe you have noticed it in someone else when you asked them why they did something? Even when the intention of the question may be rooted in curiosity, an instinct might believe it is necessary to advocate, not simply explain. Similarly, why questions can be posed as a hypothetical that quickly can also feel overwhelming to answer: "Why should I be the one to change when they're the one who's offended?" or "Why can't you just do it right?"

In those moments, the compassionate therapist may interject and invite further consideration of that question, even encouraging the client to answer it directly. "Let's pause on that for a moment, because that is a pretty substantial question! What if we really thought about it and reflected, because there is a why to what we do." This leans into the core intervention of compassionate contextualization, to be discussed in depth in the next few pages.

Using Relational "We" and "With" Language

Per the underlying theory of CRT, people exist in a collection of relationships. In the context of therapy, both the therapist and client are actively engaged with the perceived problem and the emotional experiences that accompany it. We are seeking to improve the relationship with the problem, distinct from ourselves or our loved ones. Over the course of therapy, we progress to offer it empathy and recognizing how it has not always been a problem.

As a clinician, we demonstrate language of "sitting with," "hovering over," or "diving into" a problem. This can convey the type of interactive relationship a client can have with the problem as they build their own comfort and resilience to interact with it compassionately and directly. When we are more guarded or uncomfortable being direct about the problem, we may use the more distanced language of *hovering*, shifting to *sit with* as the client learns to coexist with the problem, and *diving in* once the empathy for the problem is present.

Parts Language

Like metaphors, clients often innately use parts language about themselves: "It's like a part of me just didn't want to," or, "A part of me will always love them." CRT leans into this language because it is another way that people make sense of themselves, finding a way for multiple perspectives to coexist within them at the same time, even when they seem to contradict one another. We can normalize the experience of internal conversations all day.

In those internal conversations, an essential component is the presence of compassion in one's self-talk about and toward oneself. It can be too easy to allow inner critics free reign in our minds. This is often under the guise of providing structure and efficiency/productivity. Unfortunately, inner critics often do this harshly, and it is ultimately futile. Similar to friend-like language, CRT demonstrates and practices talking to oneself and others with the authentic kindness and accountability we would hope to receive from a loving and safe support figure. In session, therapists may invite clients to refer back to helpful statements and acts by others who care about them and practice offering those to themselves: *"When you imagine talking to your sister about this, what would you hope she would say?"*

CRT calls this our inner companion. The clinician can offer the client language of what compassionate responses they needed at different times in their life, then practicing experientially for them to offer that to themselves in the session, such as with a hand over their heart. This can be completed both individually and with client system members present, such as a partner or family member. The goal of this is to emphasize that we do not have to wait to receive these compassionate statements from our loved ones; at the same time, we are demonstrating the helpful language to them in real time for future application.

Similarly, parts language ties in with compassionate contextualization (see below). Our inner companion can offer soothing without judgment, rooted entirely in curiosity toward self or others. Doing so is not passive permission-giving; if anything, it is nonjudgmental accountability (*"Feeling this way is understandable, and acknowledging that doesn't mean we're going to stay here"*). This language can be provided by the therapist as the client adopts it over the course of their treatment process.

Compassionate Contextualization

Compassionate contextualization is the ability to ask the client to reflect on their context to make sense of why they behave, think, or feel the way(s) they do in a situation. This can be applied toward themselves or their loved ones, both in and outside the therapy room.

Recall back in Chapter 2, when we talked about the FST perspective on context. Context considers our physical and emotional settings; past, present, and future experiences and hopes; and includes personal and systemic values, beliefs, perspectives, social roles and rules, diagnoses, mood, and many other factors that contribute to our lives. There are a few ways we can ask about this: *"When you think about your life, or even just how today has gone so far, how does it make sense this is how you feel?"*

If feelings are not the focal point, you can replace that word with *think, believe, act, behave,* or *perceived a situation.* The same could be said of any of the below processes.

If the client struggles on this direct of a reflection, we can broaden the statement: *"Maybe it's not even the details about it. What would cause anyone to act that way? What things in their day contribute to a person's behaviors? What about their life experiences overall?"*

Once a person reflects on contributing factors that led to the current outcome, the therapist can provide brief psychoeducation to normalize and validate this insight (*"Of course! That makes perfect sense!"*) and describe this as identifying a person's emotional logic. Humans do not have purely cognitive logic; consistent with postmodern perspectives on ultimate truth, CRT theorizes that all people are exposed to reality through the filter of their life experience. Therefore, it makes perfect sense that different people will have differing perspectives on the same situation. The therapist can normalize this, along with compassion for the recurring themes of human struggle, such as experiences of aging, loss, hardship, failure, confusion, fluxes in motivation and mood, and desire for connection and fulfillment.

This intervention does not stop here with the insight of validation and normalization. With this intervention, we are removing the judgment that gets in the way of change via shame or guilt. After reiterating compassion via validation or normalization, the therapist guides the client to mindfully come back to the present and do a bodily check-in. This leads to the client asking themselves, "What do I need right now? What do I feel up for doing next?" Common examples of needs in that moment can be:

- Additional validation or reiteration of the compassionate message is helpful, such as from a specific person. They might want/need a loved one or partner to understand this about them.
- To verbally process grief or anger that surfaces with this recognition, often through a verbal flow of identifying emotions, thoughts, and cyclical needs with the acknowledgement of these as they come forward.
- Bodily needs such as stretching, hydrating, allowing oneself to cry, or using the restroom.

In addition to these physical needs, compassionate contextualization includes self-soothing statements rooted in shared humanity such as, *"Having needs is human, not unreasonable."* Clients can be encouraged to create these mantras for themselves based on their personal needs and shame histories. In understanding what comes next for them, we can temporarily body-double with the clients' needs and figure out where compassion is needed next.

Circular Compassionate Contextualization

Once the clinician has observed each person's ability to offer themselves compassionate contextualization, we work toward application to others in the client system, such as a romantic partner or family member.

In relationship work, the therapist will listen for which partner volunteers their introspection and emotional vulnerability first, particularly primary emotion language. The clinician may also use emotion conjecture here to prime that language. We start with this person to demonstrate receptivity to that emotionality and vulnerability and accentuate the emotional safety of the therapy space for the client to bring that depth and emotional insight. From there, the following steps may take place:

1. Therapist offers validation to Client A, along with gratitude for sharing.
2. When Client A affirms they feel heard and understood, the therapist may pose the perspective of Client B to Client A, including underlying possible emotions, and learn if they can validate this additional perspective as understandable.
3. If they are unable to validate Client B's perspective, the therapist may offer compassion as to why that would be hard to do and reiterate that seeing the additional perspective is not necessarily agreeing with it. Repeat this process as necessary until Client A can confirm seeing Client B's perspective.
4. Once they can validate Client B's point of view, the therapist then may turn to Client B and ask, "What is it like to hear your loved one acknowledge where you are coming from, that they see your point of view and understand it?" This allows the second person to also feel heard (can be bolstered by the clinician, also).
5. Similar to before, Client B may be asked to validate Client A; if able to do so, the therapist will ask Client A the same question as in the previous step.

In this way, each person can be validated, acknowledge the other person's validation, and hear the other person's appreciation for the validation. This is an essential step before moving toward creating additional change. Precise examples of this process will be included in future chapters.

Perpetual Opportunity for Compassion

Whenever working with compassion as a therapeutic emphasis, it is common for people to struggle with this. For many people, it is more automatic to be critical or judgmental toward self, others, and toward situations. The good news is we always have the opportunity to offer compassion to ourselves, even when we fail to previously. If we look back at a time when we were not compassionate, we can currently nonjudgmentally remind ourselves of the context of that situation that might have made it difficult to be compassionate.

Even if a client lacks compassion at the time of the practice in session, we can acknowledge with nonjudgmental curiosity why it was hard to be compassionate both in the moment and at the time of the incident. This process applies the "How does it make sense?" compassionate contextualization intervention even when we have failed to previously (a statement that also normalizes the human and inevitable experience of failure – and that's okay!).

Disentangling

Disentangling is the removal and pulling apart of knots and jumbles, such as rope or hair. In CRT, disentangling is a metaphor. Have you ever had the experience of putting your laundry in a tumble dryer, and when you go back to empty it, expecting it to be done, some of the sleeves and legs and socks and drawstrings have somehow managed to get themselves into such a tangle, you aren't even sure where to begin to pull it apart? And now some of those pieces are stretched and unsymmetrical, even torn. Not only that, but the clothes you expect to be dry map still be damp or wet because they got so caught up in one another. Wow, things just didn't go as planned! It's just a mess.

That's human experience so frequently. Things just don't go according to plan, and the sweater of intention and pajama pants of significance and all the other thoughts and feelings in our heart and mind . . . it gets messy. And with that mess comes frustration, confusion, and more often than not, at least a drawstring of feeling defeated.

This intervention is about pulling those tangles apart, softly and with care for how they got there and how they will be worn from here. Items that will be untangled include:

- Linear assumptions ("If this, then that")
- Assumption of intent ("They must have wanted . . .")
- Clarifying meaning-making ("They are that way because . . .")

To describe this phenomenon, the therapist might say, *"What your brain just treated as a straight line, an obvious connection, my mind missed.*

Would you expand on that for me?" followed by identifying the in-between steps, thoughts, feelings, and beliefs that the client may have glossed over without realizing those are stops along the way mentally.

Ways a therapist may further ask for clarity on these include:

○ *"What do you hear me saying right now?"*
○ *"What connections did your brain or heart just make inside you as you heard that?"*
○ *"What does that phrase mean to you?"*

All of these questions could also be shared between members of a client system to offer curiosity to one another's perspectives, suspending emotional reactivity in one's own meaning-making.

It is normal for different people to assign different meanings to certain words and ideas, often assuming other people have the same meaning when that is not necessarily the case. For example, if I say I went to the vet's office, do you imagine that means I took my pet to the veterinarian's office, or to an office managing military veterans? It could be either one; the one you think of first will typically depend on which is more immediately relevant to you.

It is worth reiterating that people make assumptions based on previous experiences. Those experiences could be situations viewed as similar, similar personalities (even previous experiences with the same person!), or even situations you heard about elsewhere. The trap is that maintaining an assumption restricts future possibilities, such as the capacity for insight, empathy, and behavioral change. It also results in deepened influence by the other person in a way that is imagined through the assumption, not factually from the other person's voiced mindset.

Meaning-making disentangling also includes exploring the relationship we have with specific words and the ideas they entail. Therapeutic examples of disentangling meaning include ideas like marriage or having a diagnosis, meaning of roles such as what it means to be a teenager or parent, and challenging the linear assumption that having standards or opinions is the same as being judgmental.

The previously mentioned intentional language of "and" is a great place to invite introspection about dichotomies we have assumed to be true about ourselves, other people, situations, and/or our relationships. For example, you may say to yourself, "How my partner set those boundaries felt bad to me." Ask yourself, can they be both a good partner *and* someone who didn't handle boundaries in a way that felt good to you? Or are they either a good partner *or* someone who can set boundaries? Can someone be a good partner but make situational missteps or cause inadvertent harm? Permitting human error without personalizing it to say something about them or you is a helpful compassion-based reflection that allows relationships and people to be their imperfect selves with nonjudgmental curiosity and insight.

An essential knot to untangle in relational compassion is the acceptance of neutrality as a recurring attribute in life and relationships. Value frequently assumes dualistic extremes, such as being either good or bad. Challenging that assumption means accepting most of life is somewhere in between. So much of day-to-day lives are unremarkable, and that's okay! Life is also remarkable – beautiful and wonderful, difficult and drudging. Neutrality is a nonthreatening reality distinct from apathy. Accepting this allows us to give ourselves and our relationships a pass on constant significance – sometimes something just *is, and* we can still grow from here.

The goal of this intervention is to step back into objectivity and look at the situation impassionately, using nonjudgmental curiosity:

- What is the belief associated with this assumption? (Could be belief[s] about oneself, another person, a situation, and/or a relationship)
- What in my history has led me to believe this belief is true?
- What about this belief has been important to me? What about it still is, or what has changed?
- What value is this assumption/belief tied to?

In many ways, this intervention is an expansion of compassionate contextualization. It nonjudgmentally makes sense of why we believe or value something and shift focus to the mindful of having a relationship with that belief. It leads to the next line of questioning: "What difference does it make to shift this perspective, or consider other possibilities?" This openness to alternatives indicates the possible presence of compassion for past perspectives (you don't have to stubbornly hold on to unhelpful ideas just because they used to work, nor do you have to be upset with yourself for them no longer working) and future options. Relationally, this question could also be, "*What changes when you assume your fellow person (partner, family member, etc.) is not the enemy, but a friend?*"

Positive Restorations

This intervention intentionally draws on the gratitude and hope rooted in positive events, views, and interactions from the past and present. It is an alternative to becoming cognitively or emotionally consumed by the negative aspects of our lives. It is not about ignoring hardships; it is more about viewing them in balance. The human mind is so good at remembering hurts; we can benefit from intentional focus on positive presences.

At this point, I can imagine the reader thinking, "Wow, 'be grateful' as an intervention? Really?" And yes, really! But maybe not the way you're expecting. We have to acknowledge (with some frustration) how popular psychology has hijacked this concept. Gratitude has sunk to be another item on the self-care list of demands, something that seems more about the check mark for completing than the practice itself. However, we're going for something very different here. It is more than a social media post about finding the sunny silver lining on a dark cloud, and it sure is distinct from toxic positivity messages to set aside uncomfortable emotions in favor of others' comfort. We're talking about creating a headspace to harmonize gratitude, lack of control, *and* personal accountability for meaningful change. Gratitude for what is can coexist with both suffering and hope for better. Here are a few ways to do that:

Peaceful Pauses

This practice is the closest CRT has to meditative practices. Take a slow, deep breath. Ask yourself, "What is good *right now?*"

The answer could be as substantial as a lengthy, constructive, heartfelt conversation with a loved one. It equally can be as temporary as a sip of your latte that was the perfect balance of flavor, texture, and temperature. They are not comparisons. Both are good. There is good in a moment. Acknowledging such does not erase the hardships; it recognizes their coexistence. And in a world where happiness, like all emotions, is temporary, acknowledging it when it happens is an essential step in experiencing joy in life.

Personal Check-Ins

An alternative to lengthier journaling assignments or bullet journals, this check-in focuses on identification of client strengths from the day and hopes for the next. It is suggested to complete this in writing, such as in a daily planner, though reflecting on it at all is helpful. Additionally, it makes the most sense to complete near the end of the day, such as part of one's sleep hygiene routine. This check-in consists of three questions:

- What is something I did today that contributed to it going well at all, even a little bit or for a little while?
- What is something today for which I can offer myself some grace?
- What is a hope I have for tomorrow?

Clients may choose to track additional information, such as their mood, medication intake, physical movement, or other information they consider relevant (self-led compassionate contextualization!).

This practice is not about the therapist asking if the client completed the task. The in-session follow-up is about the client's emotional experience and noticed changes in themselves since practicing this, regardless of frequency or thoroughness. This way, focus is on the process and benefit of reflecting on these questions, not their specific answers or the check mark of completion to appease the therapist.

Relationship Check-Ins

Like the personal check-in, this activity is meant to be completed individually and potentially reviewed together. Also similarly, it is recommended to complete as the day winds down and to possibly write down in the interest of reflection, though this is not required. For this reflection, there are four recommended questions:

- What is something about [other's name] or something they did that helped today be better, even just a little bit or for a little while?
- What is something each of us did well today?
- What is something today for which I can offer [other person] some grace?
- What is a hope I have for tomorrow, individually and/or in this relationship?

These questions hope to emphasize positive attributes in the relationship that may otherwise be overlooked. At first, it is common for the questions to require focused reflection of the previous day. Over time, people may find they think about these questions throughout the day. As a result, they notice their answers more as they occur, even identifying those positive moments to one another as they occur. This builds a greater sense of appreciation and relationship safety as the validation occurs more consistently and authentically.

Relationship Reflections: When Compassion is Missing

There are two forms of this in-session intervention, and each is broken into two parts.

The first is for when the client system comes in more emotionally heightened or describing a recent interaction that lacked compassion and was rooted in feeling unheard or misunderstood.

To begin, the therapist will offer compassion to all parties present, including identifying their perspective and offering emotional conjecture. This is a specific version of circular compassionate contextualization, with the therapist exemplifying to and teaching the client to respond with warmth when they share. In the first stage, the therapist models a compassionate affirming response; in the second stage, the partner provides that response.

Once all members of the client system in session feel heard by the therapist, we shift to focus on the stressing situation they presented with, specifically reflecting on a time when the person attempted to be compassionate toward the other person but missed the mark:

1. Identify the situation (your perspective of it).
2. Identify what you tried and the intended message.
3. Provide personal context: If this is the case, identify contributing contexts that made being compassionate in that situation difficult at that time (situational, not personal).
4. Take accountability: Offer a phrase of accepting one's role in the exchange, such as, "That being said, I recognize I missed the mark in how I said that."
5. Speculate on the other person's context: Identify what may have made receiving the message or compassion difficult in that moment for the other person, including how it makes sense why the impact would mismatch the intent. Doing this offers the other person compassion here and now about this previous miscommunication with language of shared responsibility instead of blame, which aids in present reconnection.

With the preface that the other person would likely describe the situation differently from their perspective, check in with the person receiving this. They may then go through the same sequence from their perspective, including the therapist potentially weaving in overlapping attributes from the previous version, as well.

In part two of this reflection process, we are reflecting and refocusing on a time when their system member (partner, family member) *was* compassionate to them:

1. Identify the situation (your perspective of it).
2. Verbalize your emotions and contextual history of those to your person, offering vulnerable emotional insight to yourself.
3. Identify how the other person responded that conveyed their compassion at the time, how this was helpful, and current appreciation for this response.
4. Give space for the other person to receive this reflection now, including context for how it may be both good and uncomfortable (which is okay).

If willing and emotionally safe to do so, the individuals may be encouraged to holds hands or physically touch and make eye contact while engaging in this compassionate reflection.

Relationship Reflections: When Compassion is Progressing

Once the foundation of compassion is more established, this version intentionally reiterates compassion and appreciation between client system members. These are frequently paced at about one question per session at first, but with practice, they can go faster as the mindset and language become more natural. First comes emotional-based relational reflections:

- *"When was a time this week you felt <u>connected with</u> the other person(s)?*
- *"When was a time this week you felt <u>seen/understood by</u> the other person(s)? What did they do, say, or express that gave you this feeling?"*
- *"When was a time this week you felt <u>appreciated by</u> your person(s)?"*
- *"When was a time this week you felt <u>grateful for</u> your person(s)?"*
- *"When was a time you saw your person(s) <u>needed grace</u> this week?"*

Each of these questions can be answered by each person before moving to the next, pausing between each one to hear from the other(s) what it is like to receive these acknowledgments of effort. These questions frequently overlap with compassionate contextualization, and the therapist can highlight the *both/and* component (relationship challenges and strengths).

Next, we begin the second part, the future-based relational reflections:

- "What is something you are looking forward to this week?"
- "What is something you are worried or uncertain about this week, such as a specifically demanding day or task?"
- "How can your partner offer you support this week around that worry or uncertainty?"
- "What is something you hope your partner knows about you going into this next week?"

These questions invite the clients to offer opportunities for preemptive compassion and potential insight for needed support behaviorally and compassionately. In this way, the client system begins to both offer and receive compassion directly from one another in real time.

Conversational Pauses

Both in and out of session, there can come a point when a conversation no longer feels constructive. This happens when both parties are stuck in their own perspective and unable to see the other person's. At that point, either person may request a pause or timeout (or other selected phrase or word).

This pause is not solely to go and reregulate ourselves physically. When I was growing up, sometimes I would get in fights with my sibling, and we would be sent to our rooms. This was not solely to be a punishment, it was also a time to reflect. There was not a designated length of time for this; instead, either of us could come out when we were ready to talk with our mother about our role in what happened and say sorry.

In CRT, this intentional slowdown includes some similar practices during the pause. To start, after the pause is requested, each person goes to a place they can reregulate at first. This could be going for a walk, spending time with pets, completing a task or chore, completing a brief game or puzzle, or even passive activities such as reading or watching a short video. Once your heart rate has returned to standard and you can take a few deep, slow breaths, ask yourself the following questions:

1. How does it make sense I am feeling this way?
2. What underlying belief, value, or part of me is feeling unheard or uncared for?
3. What do I need right now to offer compassion and comfort to myself? (Complete this to the best of your ability independently)
4. Knowing what I know about my loved one, how does it make sense that this is significant to them? What underlying belief, value, or part of them might be feeling unheard or uncared for?

After a standard agreed length of time (typically anywhere from 30–60 minutes), the pair can come back together and, before either restates their perspective, offer their insights to the other person's possible point of view and allow any other clarifying context the person wants to add. This practice is an essential bookend to the conflict rather than avoiding the conversation once deescalated ("Hey, what do you want for dinner?").

Temporary Agreements

Temporary agreements directly contradict some social assumptions that once a rule is established or agreement is made, it is written in stone, unchangeable. However, the nature of life and humanity includes the inevitability of change. Circumstances flux consistently; people get sick, grow, graduate, gain and lose jobs, and those are just normal life transitions. Temporary agreements also contradict the perception that the result of a disagreement must be "your way," "my way," or even mutually mediocre middle ground. It is a variation of compromise, an agreement to try something different in a few ways, for a specified durations of time, and to "live as if" for that window of time.

The goal is not to agree but to recognize there is enough safety in the relationship for the situation to be nonthreatening: "*We are designing a situational or soft agreement. What we agree to try right now doesn't have to be what we do next time. We can give ourselves the compassion to know it's okay to edit the arrangement and to do some trial and error here.*" Part of this process may include disentangling the meaning each person has about changing their minds or changing practices. For example, believing doing different than our parents must mean they were bad parents, or we were previously bad parents for the practices we used to do when less informed. Now that we know better, we can do better.

A key question when designing a temporary agreement is, "*What are the emotional needs of the outcome?*" This informs the underlying goal and formerly unmet need.

Conclusion

In addition to the interventions of metaphors, cognitive-behavioral, and compassion-, solution-, and emotion-focused therapies along with those of Satir's experiential modality, CRT brings five interventions that specifically focus on compassion as a relational game-changer. Some may start as skills, such as changing one's language to use "and" instead of "but," the purpose of these interventions is to change our relationship with our state of life through increased sense of hope and decreased personalization with improved neutrality toward hypothetical "why" questions. Similarly, compassionate contextualization is the intentional act of self-kindness rather than judgment by offering yourself understanding that you did what was understandable in a given context and it does not have to have more significant meaning than that as we address current needs. Through identifying and disentangling assumptions and meaning-making, we can also see the context behind those thoughts and emotions, furthering the compassion to be offered there. We then fold in strengths language all the more with positive restorations as intentionally positive interactions with others and oneself where these may previously have been lacking. Lastly, temporary agreements reiterates permission for the temporary to remain valid and productive, averting away from all-or-nothing perceptions of change and challenging the assumption that changes must be everlasting to be meaningful.

Chapter 6

Individuality in CRT

CRT's view of individual psyche is rooted in what we will call *social constructivism*, an integration of social constructionism and constructivism. Social constructionism theorizes one's sense of reality is learned through social observation and direct experience. Since before we can remember, we have taken in information from our surroundings. We then analyze this data to determine what is normal, designing our beliefs and values, perceptions of problems, and methods of solution-seeking and innovation. (These were also covered in Chapter 2.)

Perceptions of reality and truth are collectively created, maintained, and potentially shaped by social systems such as communities, governments, religions, and sources of education. With the internet and increased globalization, the range of these voices and messages expands worldwide. It also includes direct interactions, such as our microsystemic relationships of families, friends, teachers, and peer groups. Similar to circular causality, social constructionism is bidirectional. Individuals receive, interpret, and incorporate the information acquired from their social relationships. They also contribute to how those are maintained or amended in future relationships (sub- and suprasystems) and generations (the chronosystem).

Social constructionism is somewhat different from constructivism, which focuses on one's internal, personal, and cognitive meaning-making of one's observations and experiences. This is influenced by both social construction and brain chemistry, which influences a person's psychological flexibility and neurochemical balances. In theory, by knowing something, we can never return to a state of not knowing. Now we must either assimilate the information into our existing understanding of the functioning of the world, or restructure our understanding. In therapy, this looks like the exploration of one worldview and possible others. CRT, we call this perspective conjecture (*"What else could be true?"*).

Together, constructivism and constructionism are the internal and external contributions to identity development and one's relationships. Combined, they also circularly create and influence mental health symptomology.

DOI: 10.4324/9781003518730-7

View of Individual Symptomatology

Put simply, CRT believes there is a circular dynamic between symptoms and sources of non-optimal mental health; they are both "the chicken and the egg." At some point, we have to stop wondering which comes first and focus on how it is being perpetuated instead.

Let's reiterate the nonpathologizing stance here. Systemic therapies like CRT do not oppose the existence/influence of diagnoses; it recognizes relationships and worldviews influence and are influenced by our symptomatology. Mental health diagnoses are often defined by their symptoms, including longevity and severity. When and to what extent symptoms manifest impacts the choice of diagnosis and, potentially, one's personality.

Sources of Symptoms

It feels heavy handed to say CRT sees the source of symptoms to be one's context. As a quick refresher from Chapter 2, our context is the physical, social, and emotional settings of our emotional logic. All behavior makes sense in context. Context answers the question, "When I think about my life (or a particular action, thought, or feeling, such as a symptom of unwellness), how does it make sense?" As you might recall, this is the core question in compassionate contextualization leading to decreased judgment.

A few significant factors of past context can be:

- Who did this person look up to in childhood?
- How has this person experienced trauma or neglect throughout their life?
- What was their economic status growing up? How did they experience or view stability?
- What formal and informal education has this person received throughout life?
- What did this person learn to prioritize early in life?
- What communities did they grow up in, such as religious groups, shared interest clubs or sports teams, or extended family?

In the present, here are a few more considerations:

- Does this person feel physically and emotionally safe?
- Has this person's physical needs been met, such as consistent access to food, shelter, or healthcare?
- Do they experience recurring stressors such as being a caregiver to a loved one, including children, or have relentless job demands?
- Do they have personal or professional ambitions in life?
- What is their perception of compassion as a concept?

In addition to past and present contexts, there are internal and external sources of symptoms. External factors can include:

o Decisions of others, such as someone's substance use or family distress or disorganization, including trauma, abuse, and neglect
o Life events of circumstance, such as natural disasters, miscarriage, or unexpected financial costs
o Macrosystemic frustration, such as cost of living, legal decisions, systemic discrimination and injustice

Internal sources of symptomology can be cognitive ("mind") or physical ("brain"):

o Mismatch between expectations and reality
o Past experiences and meaning given to these
o "Illusion of control" over areas of concern and influence (see Chapter 2)
o Physical health, including chronic illness and acute medical stressors
o Brain structure and neurochemicals

Let's talk more about that last item. Biologically, mental health diagnoses are an outcome of brain structure and effectiveness of neurochemicals in the brain. Neurochemicals include serotonin, dopamine, epinephrine, norepinephrine, endorphins, glutamate, gamma-aminobutyric acid (GABA), histamine, and glycine. In various combinations, neurotransmitters impact mood, sleep, metabolism, sexual health, nervous and cardiovascular systems, and executive functioning (focus and alertness, memory, decision-making, sensory processing, motivation). Brain structure can be more permanent and result in symptoms tied to neurodevelopmental disorders. At the time of writing this book, these are colloquially referred to as *neurodivergence*.

Neurodiversity and Neurodivergence

Neurodiversity is the whole range of human neurological functioning, including behavioral traits, cognitive habits, and emotional patterns. Approximately 15–20% of individuals are believed to be neurodiverse. This covers numerous diagnoses including autism spectrum disorder (ASD); learning disorders; attention and impulsivity disorders; and anxiety disorders such as social anxiety, sensory processing, and obsessive compulsive disorder (OCD).

Neurodivergence is when one's mental functioning is considered outside the society's idea of what is "typical," or normal. Brains that function in a way that works well in a specific culture/environment are called *neurotypical*. However, "normal" is socially constructed, subjective, and often rooted in assumptions of a narrow definition of optimal functioning in a specific societal structure. Even if we say it's what's most common, it tends to be tied to what is common for a certain population, usually the population in power.

Instead, think of it as a spectrum. If we put functioning within a society on one axis, and functioning within oneself on another, there is one corner that is optimal functionality in both. The further someone is from that ideal, the more influential their symptoms are likely to be in their lives. Similar to mindful self-compassion (MSC), CRT works well with neurodivergence to decrease personalization and self-criticism or self-judgment. MSC research shows high benefit to parents of children with ASD, too, through improving emotional openness, improving self-kindness and self-forgiveness, better time management, increased parenting confidence, and decreased sense of guilt over mistakes. Key factors contributing to these reportedly include knowledge of the diagnosis (psychoeducation!), social support and understanding, and internal resources to challenge unrealistic expectations. CRT would call this disentangling and compassionate contextualization.

CRT is Neurodiverse Affirming

Per the CRT perspective, a person's neurodivergence is not something to be fixed. It is not, by itself, viewed as the problem. If anything, the assumption that it is the problem is part of the problem. As was said earlier in this section, the relationship with the symptom or source – including your brain – is where both problems and potential solutions sit. Working with neurodiverse populations means looking for what works best for them to optimize their functioning within the range of social suitability.

I have had clients struggle with that last statement, asking why it is their responsibility to shift into a socially suitable version of themselves. To this I say, you're right, it isn't fair in a lot of ways. But where we can't shift the circle of concern, we can shift the circle of control. A big part of this with clients is differentiating masking and coping.

- *Masking* is when people conceal or suppress their neurodiverse qualities, often bending to social pressures to gain social acceptance. This is something all people do to an extent, moderating their behavior in some settings, such as having a "phone voice" or behaving more extraverted in a customer service job. Masking becomes problematic when it is ongoing, often resulting in increased anxiety, depression, and lost sense of self. It is often steeped in shame and pressure to pretend to appear neurotypical for the comfort of others.

- *Coping*, on the other hand, is gaining tools to use one's unique strengths and communication skills to discover and live the optimal version of yourself. These help neurodiverse people coexist with neurotypical expectations. This can include mental and behavioral skills for self-advocacy and self-care.

Neurodivergent-Mindful CRT Interventions

Ideally, CRT helps clients love their neurodiverse-ness as a part of them while also holding that it is not their whole self. They can take care of that part, event molding aspects of their life to take care of it, such as through job choice (Don't work in a call center if talking on the phone is a huge source of anxiety, for example) and finding what works for them in daily life structure and decision (wardrobe, time management, etc.).

In CRT, the key is compassion as a balance of kindness and accountability. Usually masking and other symptoms are maladapted responses to a previously needed survival mechanism. If we can offer that part compassion, not judgment or criticism, symptoms tend to be more receptive to conversations of change, demonstrating cognitive flexibility. Self-acceptance is not passivity toward a diagnosis or symptoms; it is not saying, "It's fine to avoid this because I have . . ." Instead, CRT differentiates masking and coping, using compassionate contextualization is a coping skill unto itself (*"How does it make sense this tool helps?"*). We can also offer self-soothing statements (*"It's ok to use tools. It would be unrealistic to expect someone to never need them. It is normal to use more of what works."*).

Diagnoses, including but not limited to neurodivergence, can also be an opportunity to disentangle the relationship people have with a diagnosis, theirs or a loved one's:

- *"What does it mean to have that label?"*
- *"What do you believe it says about the symptom-bearer to be diagnosed?"*
- *"How does everyone view their relationship with the diagnosis, distinct from the symptom-bearer?"* (Remember, there is more to a person than their diagnoses)
- *"What does it mean to intentionally work with, not against/despite, with the diagnosis?"*

So, How Does Change Happen Individually?

The good news is that the extent of symptomology and intrusiveness thereof is highly malleable. They can be altered with cognitive and behavioral changes, including how we think and treat our emotional health. This is the emphasis of CRT – the change comes from how we interact with our problems, decreasing shame and increasing compassion toward self and others. Research has shown our neurochemical balances are not static; what we do and how we think and feel impact them, circular with how our neurochemicals impact us.

Remember, a key perspective in CRT that differentiates it from other modalities is that we believe people have a relationship with the diagnosis and one's symptoms. You have feelings about your anxiety, lack of motivation, paranoia, proneness to personalize or exaggerate, and so on. How you feel about them impacts how they present, but hating them and wishing they weren't there does not, in fact, make them go away. In fact, sometimes it seems to make them cling on tighter. I imagine our symptoms are like children eager to please a trusted adult. When they upset that adult and the adult turns away, the child holds on all the more, fearful of losing their relationship with that trust figure.

Therefore, with any presenting problem, CRT approaches the conversation from the lens of healing the relationship with the diagnosis or symptoms. The goal is to decrease the stress associated with the symptom. If this results in a lessening of some symptoms, that is not assumed to be good or bad. Paradoxically, you can't go into this practice hoping for the symptom to go away; as odd as it may be, it's like the symptom can sense when that's the case, and goes back to clinging on. Instead, we seek to understand the positive purpose or misunderstanding of the symptom that makes it behave as it does. When we approach parts of ourselves with kindness and mindfulness rather than criticism, they are more receptive to change. In this way, even in individual therapy, CRT continues to use relational methods to heal.

Modality Comparison: Cognitive Behavioral Therapy

Like CRT, Cognitive Behavioral Therapy (CBT) works with the overlap between thoughts and behaviors (and emotions, though this comes later in CBT) and overall wellbeing, noticing that change in one can create change in the other two. This can be true both in the individual and between people, influencing one another. Both models of therapy look at automatic or intrusive thoughts, which CBT calls cognitive distortions, that result from linear assumptions and faulty meaning-making. These include overgeneralizing; black/white thinking; minimizing or magnifying; mind-reading; or personalization. Mindful self-compassion calls the latter the antithesis of shared humanness, and is key in CRT.

CBT is known for their intervention of cognitive restructuring, which challenges the validity of previous thought patterns. One way to do this is to have people attempt to defend their perspective within themselves or with others. If the defense is deemed insufficient, it is declared invalid and rejected. In theory, this helps someone be more grounded in reality rather than fear. Personally, that hurts my heart. The intentional invalidation and rejection of one's thoughts and feelings may perpetuate old norms of emotional suppression, not emotion regulation. As I once had a client say, "it seems like gaslighting yourself."

Most substantially, an essential key difference between CRT and CBT is the perception of emotional logic, or emotional reasoning. CBT considers emotional logic to be problematic, rooted in reactivity, defiling true reality. CRT embraces emotional logic as our experience of reality. It is the flawed, human logic that always makes sense in context. To grant yourself this compassion allows the interventions that come after to be more effective in improving our relationships.

CRT Interventions in Individual Therapy

To demonstrate the use of CRT interventions with an individual client, let's use a case example. Johanna is a 36-year-old second-generation Indian woman who has lived in the United States since her parents immigrated there when she was around five years old. When I first met Johanna, she said she wanted therapy to help her cope with feeling overwhelmed all day, every day, and she wanted to "actually like herself . . . for the first time in [her] life."

In our first meeting, I learned that she had previously been married to Dominic, a white 44-year-old man, and they shared custody of their two children, Olivia (12F) and Isaiah (9M). About two years ago, she married Lexi, who is 38 years old and nonbinary, whom she met through a dating app. She lists out problem after problem in each of these relationships, not to mention stress at her job as an administrator at a medical office. As Johanna spewed about these stressors, I barely had to ask questions; she was so eager to have someone to talk to about her struggles. At the end, she sighed and said, "So tell me what to do, Doc. Tell me how to fix it." I chuckled a little, suspecting she would not be entirely pleased with my reply.

"Well, Johanna, the good news is your stress about these is completely understandable. I felt the tiredness and overwhelm even as you shared it! And I hear so many pieces that seem to feel so out of your control, which is a whole exhaustion unto itself." She nods adamantly. "That being said, I imagine it is even scarier to consider that not only do you *feel* out of control of so much, you *can't* control so much." She freezes and looks down at her lap. "What happens for you when I say that? What just went through your mind and heart?"

This was the beginning for Johanna and I as we began to pull apart her linear assumptions, harsh self-talk, and sources of her relationship struggles. Below are snippets of our conversations that demonstrate CRT interventions in action.

Intentional Language

When discussing Johanna's view of herself, here is an example of and/but language:

Therapist:	"You mentioned in our first meeting that you want to like yourself. What would be different when you liked yourself?"
Johanna:	"Well, I wouldn't second-guess myself all the time. And I wouldn't be so self-critical, like, all the time, but I just don't seem to be able to help it."
T:	"I could see that making a big difference for anyone! It sounds like that self-critical part of you has really been influential for a while?"
J:	"Oh, absolutely."
T:	"How do you feel about that self-critical part of you?"
J:	"She's awful. I wish she would just go away."
T:	"Wow. I imagine as you said that, that self-critical space inside you just dug their heels into your brain that much more."
J:	[chuckling] "Yea, probably."
T:	"It reminds me of when a child anticipates their parent is mad at them, right? How did you respond to your parents' emotions when you were younger?"
J:	"Oh, I completely shut down. My mom was very sensitive. I usually ended up comforting her and calming her down.
T:	"Wow, that's a lot of responsibility on a child, to take care of a parent. That sounds like it would have been really challenging."
J:	[becoming tearful] "I think it was, but she was a great mom."
T:	"What does the critical part of you say about her?"
J:	"That she tried as hard as she could."
T:	"I wonder how it would feel for us to recognize both? That yes in a lot of ways she was a great mom, and also we were in a really tough position trying to take care of a parent?
J:	"I guess so. [pause] I never thought of it that way."

Compassionate Contextualization

When discussing Johanna's relationship with her children, here's an example of initiating compassionate contextualization:

Therapist: "It sounds like it feels really discouraging to you when you tell your kids they need to do their homework after school, and they just ignore you. You try and ask nicely, and it's like they don't acknowledge you at all. It's only when Lexi threatens to take their tablets away that they respond at all, and even then, it's begrudgingly. Is that a fair summary?"

Johanna: "Unfortunately, yea. And after a long workday, I just don't have the energy for it."

T: "I imagine so! Being in charge of another human's behavior is so hard and can feel unwinnable. Answer this for me. When you look back at how you were raised, or when you and Dom were together, how does it make sense that it is so hard for you to get your kids to do what you tell them?"

J: "I mean, because they're kids. They want to get away with whatever they can."

T: "Hmm. And how does it make sense that would be discouraging for you?"

J: "Well, when I was growing up, Pappa's word was law. If he told you to do something, you dropped whatever you were doing before and did what he asked, right then and there. That's what we were taught to do.

T: "How scary I imagine that feels to not know what happens there. Another example of feeling discouraged, maybe?"

J: "Absolutely!"

T: "What other words or emotions does your brain tie to parenting?"

J: "Hmm. Probably overwhelming. Frustrating. Lonely. Which isn't fair to Lexi; I know she does so much."

T: "That's ok; it is an honest feeling. I wonder if you'll try something with me right now. Would you mind sitting back, [slow the pace of speech], placing your hand on your heart, and taking a deep breath in through your nose, pause a moment, and exhale with a sigh."

Johanna does these steps as I describe them.

T:	"And with your hand over your heart, offer to yourself, out loud or in your head, the statement, 'I am feeling discouraged with how parenting is going. It is understandable I feel that way when I feel overwhelmed or frustrated, too. I was raised different. I try so hard, and it doesn't go the way I hope. It makes so much sense that would feel discouraging." *We pause while Johanna sits in silent, nodding slowly with mild tearfulness.*
T:	"I wonder what your heart and soul need right now? What's happening inside you right this moment?"
J:	"It just feels . . . so much. Relieving. Sad. Confusing because I still want to do differently."

Disentangling

This is a sample of disentangling meaning-making and linear assumptions regarding Johanna's self-perception tied to self-worth:

Therapist:	"You've described so many sources of stress in your life, both in the past and right now. What does that critical part of you believe it says about you that you are overwhelmed by all these stressors coming together?"
Johanna:	"Well, I don't think it says anything about me personally, but I still feel like I should be able to just figure it out and handle it. I feel like I used to be able to."
T:	"That's good that you are able to not take that to heart! It is human nature to feel overwhelmed when stressors seem to outweigh our capacities. When you look back on your life, where did you learn how much you should be able to handle?"
J:	"Um, well, I don't know. I guess I always saw my parents able to handle whatever life threw at them, you know?"
T:	"That makes perfect sense. From what you saw, they could handle everything that got thrown at them. From the outside, I bet it looked like they really knew what they were doing, huh?"
J:	"Oh, my father was the king of making things look easy."

> T: "So maybe there's an assumption about what you 'should' be able to handle based on what you observed as a kid in your parents, and also a recognition now, as an adult, that your view back then may have been limited?"
>
> J: "Yea, that's true. I don't actually know they handled everything well; I'm assuming that they did."
>
> T: "And maybe, therefore, that "should" is a bit biased in its perspective, too?"
>
> J: "Yea, I could see that. It makes me feel a little better. Some of the judgment comes off."

Positive Restorations

When discussing Johanna's self-compassion, here's an example of a positive restoration personal check-in, in session:

> Therapist: "In our last session, we talked about you trying that brief pseudo-journaling practice of just answering those three questions once a day or at night: What is something I did today that contributed to it going well at all, even a little bit or for a little while? What is something today for which I can offer myself some grace? And what is a hope I have for tomorrow? How did that go?"
>
> Johanna: "Well I didn't do it every night like I wanted to, but I did it a few times."
>
> T: "And what did you notice felt different those nights or the days after, even just a little?"
>
> J: "I noticed I could relax a little better and maybe fell asleep faster?"
>
> T: "Wow! It sounds like it helped you feel more calm as you wound down your day."
>
> J: "Yea, and a few days, I found myself thinking about it during the day. Like the other day, I was dealing with a customer at work who was just being so rude, and I was able to stay calm and not take it personally. Afterwards, my supervisor told me she overheard me and told me

> | T: | good job. In that moment, I thought to myself, 'This could be the thing I did that helped my day go well.'" |
> | --- | --- |
> | T: | "So even in the moment, you started being able to give yourself credit for things you were doing well. That's amazing. What a shift!" |

A note to readers, notice that the therapist does not ask for the content of what she contributed or what she gave herself grace for. The focus is on the process and experience of the grace and self-recognition.

Temporary Agreements

When discussing Johanna's plan to talk to her wife about their relationship, here's an example of laying out a temporary agreement:

Johanna:	"I really wish Lexi would come to counseling with me sometime. I think it would do us good."
Therapist:	"How has it been to talk to her about that?"
Johanna:	"She's hesitant, I think. She says she wants to feel more connected with me but doesn't believe talking to a stranger about it is the way to make it happen." [chuckles]
T:	"I could see that. Therapy can seem strange to people who are used to keeping their problems to themselves, even when doing that is exactly part of what keeps us stuck sometimes."
J:	"Exactly!"
T:	"How have the two of you connected in the past, even just a little bit or for a little while?"
J:	"We used to go out more. Little concerts or local comedy shows, that sort of thing. Sometimes we'd just go walk around the park near the kids' school."
T:	"What would it be like to invite her on a walk once a week for the next month or so? Maybe on one of the nights the kids are with their dad?"
J:	"Oh, I don't think she'd want to make that part of the routine. She likes to get stuff done on the nights the kids are gone with their dad."

T: "It doesn't have to be a forever routine. The hope is a brief reminder of what that reconnection feels like. And if the month passes and it doesn't help, we can try something different. That's ok. That is still the two of you growing and figuring things out together."

J: "I could try that. I think she'd feel better if I put it that way."

Part II

Family Therapy Application

Chapter 7

Compassionate Relational Family Therapy

Some early forms of FST overlook compassion's role in interactive components of relationships. CRT with families provides language and tools to teach adults the compassion to break cycles of generational or personal trauma. We will talk more about trauma in Chapter 15. For now, we focus on family-based compassionate interventions through resilience-building, validation and normalization, and shifting language to allow change led by love and compassion.

Family as Source of Resilience

A growing body of research shows that relational support and resilience are more indicative of future quality of life than the number of adverse childhood experiences (ACEs) early in life. Lately, resilience as a concept has gotten a rough reputation, akin to the need to "be strong" in the face of adversity, often assumed via toxic positivity or emotional callousness. However, we view it differently; it is simply the ability to adapt and overcome. Of course we wish this wasn't a necessary skill; it is exhausting (arguably impossible) to be consistently resilient! However, this is exactly where family can step in as a guide and source of support. To do this, CRT psychoeducation references two systemic perspectives that highlight the potentially positive impact of family in how people cope with change: the Circumplex and ABC-X Models.

Circumplex Model

Family is where we learn how to connect with people and adapt in situations benign, bothersome, and overbearing. The Circumplex Model concentrates on two variables that impact family stress management, each viewed as a spectrum: cohesion and adaptability.

DOI: 10.4324/9781003518730-9

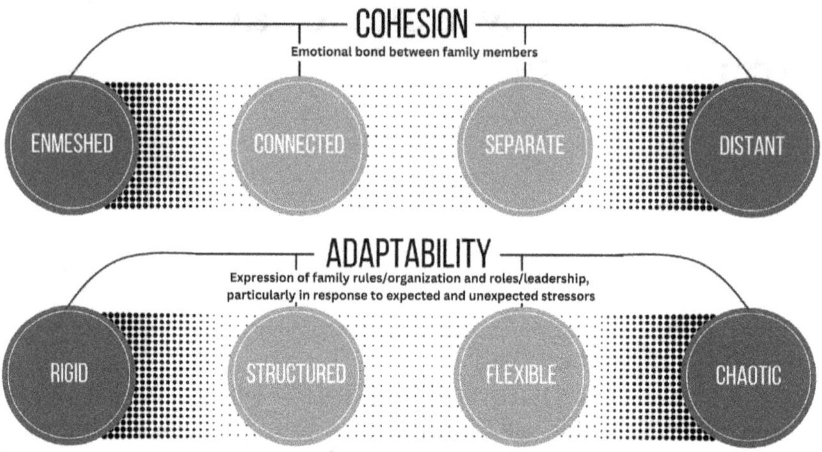

Figure 7.1 Circumplex Model Variables: Cohesion & Adaptability

Among these, connected, separated, structured, and flexible are considered balanced; enmeshed, disengaged, rigid, and chaotic are imbalanced. Putting these on a grid, the family will fall into one of sixteen categories, as seen in Figure 7.2.

The Family Adaptability and Cohesion Evaluation Scales (FACES-IV) is a self-reporting assessment tool available online that places a family in one of sixteen squares, based on each family member's perception. With this information, we can spotlight existing strengths (balanced) and potential

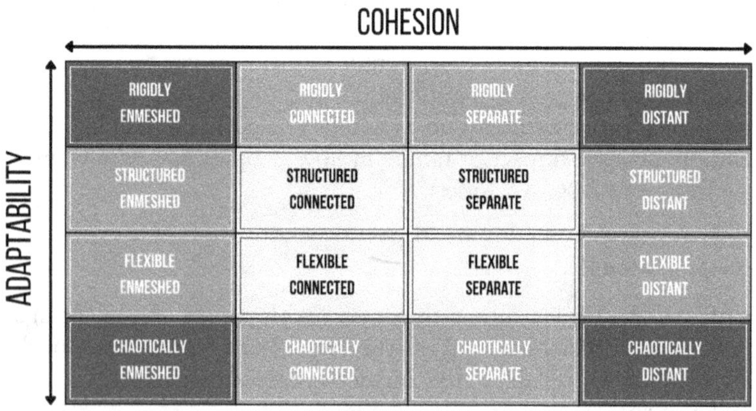

Figure 7.2 Circumplex Model: Couple and Family Map

areas of change (unbalanced). We can also compassionately reflect on how the system learned their tendencies, explore differing expectations of ideal connectedness and flexibility, and contextualize unbalanced responses as both understandable and unhelpful.

These categorizations also explain behaviors people may not realize are a reflection of cohesion and adaptability, such as:

- Strict boundary setting
- Firm hierarchical leadership roles
- Inconsistent discipline practices
- Perceptions of loyalty rooted in obedience
- Emotional volatility

Double ABC-X Model of Family Crisis and Resilience

Consistent with systemic approaches to trauma, CRT is informed by the ABC-X and its descendent, the Double ABC-X, models that looks at family crisis and resilience. The latter takes further consideration of the variables' complexities:

- A – the stressor event, the pain, or source of distress. Expanded to include the "pileup" of additional stressors that build off the original, such as financial anxiety that comes with losing a job.
- B – the existing resources, expanded to include resources newly accessible/available after the event. This includes material, emotional, and relational resources to ensure both physical and psychological needs are met.
- C – the perception of the stressor(s), resources, and oneself, along with one's relationships with those.

Together, B and C could be considered one's coping skills and capacities to adapt.

- X – the resulting extent of trauma, viewed through a spectrum of adaptability, ranging from crisis victimhood to resilient.

This model (see Figure 7.3) emphasizes the role of ongoing support and compassion (toward self and others) as both a resource and influence on perception of an event. With this approach, building resilience is the application of a soothing salve to heal a hurt, not developing a callus to dull the pain.

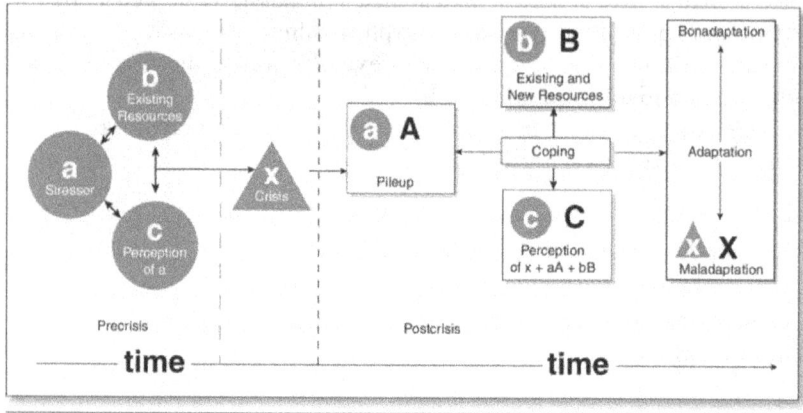

Figure 7.3 ABC-X/Double ABC-X Model

Family as Source of Validation and Normalization

Social support systems provide examples of human functioning, exemplifying how to problem-solve, adapt, and cope with that which is outside one's control. This includes teachers, coaches, counselors, extended family, and especially those in a parenting role. These leaders have the opportunity to teach essential skills of normalizing and validating, often by demonstrating these for self and others:

1. Normalize taking responsibility for one's contributions to problems and apologizing, verbally and behaviorally.
2. Normalize *not* taking responsibility for contributions from others to a problem. We can care for and support someone without being personally responsible for their wellbeing or decisions.
3. Normalize difficult moments/transitions as common life experience people can persevere through, meeting these rather than resisting them.
4. Validate relational hurt while also differentiating people and their actions. We can accept and love someone as a person without approving of their actions.
5. Validate other perspectives and view them as equally valid to one's own.
6. Set and convey clear expectations for self and others.
7. Demonstrate reasonable flexibility about positive outcomes.

These compassionate acts are particularly influential among family, where in the same setting we uniquely have meaningful horizontal relationships (defined by relational equality) and vertical (distinct in the uneven distribution of power, authority, and knowledge, often due to age differences and caregiving roles). In both structures, the "us against a problem" mentality is pivotal to working as a team without making a designated symptom bearer the problem (because we all know people are more beautifully complex than that!).

It is fair to acknowledge this may be the ideal interaction with support system; it is unfortunately common for this to not be the case. People in leadership positions can be harsh, critical, and unsupportive, often based on their previous experiences, too. These will begin to be explored early in family therapy during assessment and throughout interventions.

Family Assessment Features

In family therapy, assessment and interventions are an ongoing exchange; assessing is a form of intervention. Important assessment data to collect is the client system members' current life stages, deviations and challenges from those, and expectations of family functioning. These are in addition to the assessment questions/concepts identified earlier assessing for current capacities and perceptions of compassion. All of these fold in with psychoeducation from the therapist.

Client Life Stages

"What's your age? How do you like this age? What's nice about it? What's hard about it?"

Erik Erikson, a well-known psychoanalyst, proposed an age-based sequence of biopsychosocial developmental events. Of course, we must acknowledge this research, which began in the mid-twentieth century, is rooted in Caucasian, protestant, cis/hetero-normative, neurotypical, middle-class assumptions. With that in mind, Figure 7.4 provides a summary of those 'typical' life stages.

While Erikson's theory is more complex than this simplified table, CRT uses this as a foundation for compassionate validation of the hardships of both expected and unexpected life challenges. There are five normalizing takeaways from the theory:

1. Growth occurs across all ages; life is never static.
2. Identity includes continuity of attributes across life stages and the development of new ones over time.
3. Aspects of a person – biologically, psychologically, socially, spiritually – must be viewed in integration with one another, in the context of the environment.

Life Stage	Ages	Common Life Stage Events	Common Challenges at This Stage
Infancy	Birth – 2 years	Motor skills (grasping, pinching), causal schemes, mirroring, receptive listening, initial attachment	Physical weakness, susceptible to injury, lack verbalization, sleep disturbance, total dependence on adults for hygiene and emotional regulation
Toddlerhood	2–4 years	Improved physical coordination, mental and symbolic/fantasy play, daily vocabulary growth, initial self-regulation and empathy development	Tantrums and meltdowns (differentiated by ability to reregulate independently), aggression (biting, hitting, hair-pulling), lying, blaming language, pretending not to hear someone, picky eater, ongoing sleep disturbances
Early school age	4–6 years	High curiosity, formation of a conscience, formation of friendships and peer play, beginning of formal education	Body/sex curiosity, including masturbation and curiosity about the physical differences between people with a vagina versus penis, identification of neurological disorders (autism, ADHD, learning disorders), language limitations to express feelings, adjusting to the structure of a classroom
Middle childhood	6–12 years	Concrete operations, metacognitions and capacity for self-evaluation, skill learning (social, technical, academic), team/cooperative play	Increased risk of peer rejection and social isolation, self-evaluation rooted in social comparison with risks of misperception and high risk of personalization
Early adolescence	12–18 years	Physical maturation/puberty, introduction of romantic/sexual identity exploration, increased ability to think about logical processing and future planning	Egocentricism ("everyone thinks and lives like me"), mismatching emphasis on 'discover yourself' while also 'fitting in' with a peer group, hypersensitivity to hypocrisy, increased risk-taking/impulsive behavior, technology exposure
Later adolescence	18–24 years	Increased autonomy (self-sufficiency, self-differentiation from family of origin, distinguishing social and moral issues), synthesizing gender identity, introduction to career path	Role experimentation (trying different jobs, different interests/hobbies, varied dating practices), learning how to interact with former caregivers/mentors when no longer rooted in convenience/filial obligation; "boomerang children" (launched children returning to family of origin housing, often due to financial limits)
Early adulthood	2–34 years	Expanding roles among different settings (personal, professional), increased emphasis on finding and living one's best self; finding long-term partnerships, childbearing and childrearing, stabilizing living environment (setting 'roots' somewhere through established job or purchasing a home)	Role conflict, overload, or strain; shifting from idealized to realistic relationship expectations; choosing between cohabitation versus marriage; choosing whether or not to have children; fertility problems; increased intentionality to address sleep, nutrition, and fitness to prolong physical wellness
Middle adulthood	34–60 years	Managing a career and household (practically and finding life balance), nurturing relationships (romantic/sexual, peer, and familial), launching children	"Sandwich generation" challenges of caregiving both the younger and older generations, potentially including parent death; possible divorce and remarriage/blending families; midlife career change or loss
Later adulthoo	60–75 years	Reflecting on self, emotions, values, and situational context to problem-solve; some cognitive decline; expression of new interests/hobbies with retirement; grandparenthood; increased loss of one's peer group/partner(s)	Socialization after retirement, financial stress associated with potential retirement, changes in sexual functioning and social stigma around sexual expression as a senior, death anxiety
Elderhood	75+ years	Sensory decline; decreasing physical resilience; slowed reaction time, problem-solving abilities, memory skills, and information processing	Loss of independent functioning or living arrangements, finding motivation to continue living, grief, continued decline in physical health/strength, medical treatments and costs, lowering quality of life,

Figure 7.4 Lifespan Development Stages

4. People actively contribute to their development; we are not passive participants to life.
5. Diversity contributes to systemic enrichment, including its stability.

Throughout all stages of life, this information offers a ready-made example of self-compassion's attribute of shared human experiences: Your specific experience may be unique, and at the same time, you are not alone in your life challenges.

Deviations from Expected Life Transitions

"How has this part of life been different than you expected?"
There is a degree of flexibility in "normal" ages and life events based on cultural norms such as socioeconomic factors, religious influences, education, and collectivistic or individualistic ideals. Outside this variance, some deviations are undeniably intrusive to a sense of normalcy or functionality, long or short term:

- Out-of-order events, such as the loss of parental rights or the untimely death of a parent
- Divorce
- Gender transitions
- Child mortality
- Chronic illness
- Legal problems
- Job or housing instability
- Natural disasters

Some people may argue that many of these examples are becoming increasingly normal. Transitions, expected or not, can be complicated by confusion, grief, and a barrage of other emotions. CRT emphasizes creating space (and permission) to take time to grieve these deviations as part of adapting to them. For example, we can validate that it is common for life not to be easy or go as expected/planned, and that does not make it insurmountable. Chances are, you are not the first person to go through this specific struggle, nor will you be the last. It is hard because it is new to you; your experience of it is unique to your context, and you are not alone!

A Note from Bethany: I frequently work with LGBTQIA+ clients. When therapy is focused on their coming out and/or transitioning, an important part of my job is exploring their family's adjustment to their transition, too. This covers processing grief of the life that could have been, the complexity of past memories, and questions they may have practically (psychoeducation) or about the future of the relationship. In the interest of everyone's emotional safety, we do not directly process the family members' feelings with the transitioning individual, who is likely coping with their own. Though this is an individual's identity shift, it impacts the system, and we want to approach that mindfully.

Family Structure and Functioning

Expectations of family structure and functioning is primarily rooted in role expectations and confusion. Here are a few questions you can ask in assessment about this:

"Who lives at home?"

This can be a complicated question. There may be multiple homes due to co-parenting. A parent may be inconsistently present due to military involvement or incarceration. There may not be housing stability, such as they could be living in hotels, a vehicle, or in someone else's home. The client may not live at home, may be avoiding home or running away. Additional questions of emotions around these variations may follow.

"What do you think of when I say the phrase 'family roles'? What role(s) do you play in your life? In your family?"

In FST, roles tend to be tied to responsibilities and relationship between system members: Mother, father, step-parent, grandparent, child, and so on. Often, people unknowingly have mismatched expectations from one another of those roles. We ask about this to assess the capacity to see one another's perspectives and hardships independent of their own lens ("What is it like to see someone struggle to meet expectations of their role? What do you think contributes to that hardship?").

Virginia Satir, a foundational theorist in early family therapy, defined family roles by communication roles:

1. *Placater* – passive, highly agreeable, conflict avoidant. Tend to be anxious about how others experience them and worry taking a stance will lead to disconnect.
2. *Blamer* – combative or complacent, heavily emphasize external contributors to their problems. Often lonely.
3. *Computer* – appears unemotional, hyperrational, and more likely to treat their perception as factual. Often vulnerable underneath this shell, afraid to make mistakes or appear misinformed.

4. *Distractor* – manipulates others' emotions to avoid their own underlying uncomfortable emotions through anger, guilt, or otherwise redirecting focus off themselves.

From a compassionate lens, all four communication styles are guarded, seeking emotional safety, connection, and space for personal autonomy, too.

After describing these, a counselor may ask, *"Which of these communication styles seem most accurate to what you see yourself do?"* followed by the circular question, *"What's it like to hear one another acknowledge their imperfections or underlying emotions?"* Lastly, we can introduce the fifth role:

5. *Leveler* – emotionally balanced through compassionate self-reflection, using congruent communication (matching verbal and nonverbal cues).

From there, we can ask each person about the differences they see between what they currently do and the Leveler, including strengths-based questions of when they have seen those qualities in themselves and/or one another (*"Tell me about a time you saw Leveler qualities in your son"*).

"How do you contribute to your family? What is your 'job' there? How would you hope to be a family contributor? How do you hope others would contribute?"

This is another way of asking about the perceived function of the roles people fill. These include age- and developmentally-appropriate chores and acts of autonomy, particularly among children; financial or material contributions; home upkeep and services, such as chores; and emotional responsibilities to one another, soothing or "fixing" relational problems, such as Satir's role types. Hopefully, this will also include the eight sources of family normalization and validation identified earlier in the chapter.

As we ask about these, we must acknowledge cultural influences of these, such as at what age someone is expected to get a job and start contributing to the upkeep of the home or care for other children, or pets in the home. Clinicians can talk with clients about what is expected of them based on cultural and familial assumptions.

"What do you feel like you can't talk about with family, or specific members of the family?"

Often, systems remain in semi-functional homeostasis because certain topics, memories or parts of oneself are kept hidden or silent. This question intentionally brings those to the forefront both as a way of encouraging vulnerability and to inform the therapist of a possible covert goal: to be able to live authentically around one another. To encourage honesty, it may be beneficial to ask this question in a written initial assessment questionnaire rather than verbally asked in session, especially when rapport is still burgeoning.

To begin addressing these, family therapy may meet with subsystems periodically, such as pairs of people. The therapist may reiterate their secret-keeping policy (we will neither join in on keeping a secret nor be the spiller of secrets, instead giving space for a family member to speak the secret themselves). From there, we discuss with those subsystems what purpose the secret has in the homeostasis, the degree of urgency to share those, the difference between secrecy and privacy, and the relationship each person has with the secret and act of secret-keeping; it may feel like a moral injury, which contributes to urgency.

"What does a 'normal' family look like to you? What about 'healthy'?"

Gone are the days of assuming anyone you meet comes from a family with two biological parents married to one another, steady income, and steady housing. Instead, we must be mindful of the multitude of family structures. Each of these can contribute to role confusion, especially amidst change:

- Single parenthood – fulfilling all parent roles, such as disciplinarian, sole breadwinner, and caregiver.
- Co-parenthood – role differences between primary and secondary parents when parenting time is not split 50/50; challenges when parents are uncommunicative or hostile with one another, including for safety reasons, rather than collaborative).
- Blended families (different responsibilities as a biological or initial parent versus step-/bonus parent; multiple children in competing roles [such as two who previously were both the oldest, possibly parentified, children]; shift from being an only child; a male child who was tasked with being "the man of the house" asked to step down).
- Extended family member(s) as primary caregivers (can be confusing to family decision-making hierarchy about a child's wellbeing).
- Latchkey kids (parentified children).
- Split generational children, or large age gaps between siblings/sibling sets (varied emotional connectedness between siblings close versus distant in age).
- Adoption and foster families (can contribute to low sense of stability/permanence; difficulty developing a systemic identity when "family" may seem highly fluid/temporary or overtly unsafe).

We identify these differences because role confusion can be highly detrimental to mental peace, and compassion is essential to stabilizing. This is particularly true in the first few years of transition between these structures, regardless of age. As we ask about client definitions of normal or healthy, it is important to emphasize the emotions and felt safety of these, not only the external structure (*"When has your family aligned or been similar with that, even temporarily or situationally?"*).

Establishing Relational Treatment Goals

These questions are consistent with any client system presenting for therapy:

1. How are they hoping therapy will help them, individually and in their relationship?
2. How do they hope their relationship will look different, which would show therapy was constructive?
3. What do they hope they will be doing/thinking/feeling differently when therapy is done?

Specific to family systems, it is important to get these answers from each person in attendance. Additionally, the therapist can use this as a launching point to demonstrate validation and synthesize goals to highlight how each person's goals overlap with one another's, such as emphasizing a shared interest in feeling safe around one another, to know how they fit in one another's lives, and wanting to be understood in times of stress.

Noticing Aloud in Family Assessment

Throughout the first few sessions, it can be particularly significant to notice not only the interactions of attendees but a few other observations:

- Who is present? Absent? (*"I notice oldest brother is not here."*)
- Where is it hard to offer compassion? (*"I notice it seems particularly hard to validate Dad's addiction. I wonder if that's because it seems impossible to validate without it seeming to say the way he acted while drunk was ok, or that he yelled at Mom was ok."*)
- Who gets triangulated? (Hint! It might be you.) (*"I noticed when he said he wanted to buy a new truck, you turned toward me, waving your hand at him, and said, 'See what I have to deal with?'"*)

Intervention Applications and Case Example

In Chapter 6, we introduced Johanna. She came to therapy to work through feelings of overwhelm. As we talked with her, we learned about the people around her who influence her mental health, and she influences theirs! If we worked with her family instead of just her, here are some examples of how the key interventions might look:

Intentional Language

Early in their marriage, Johanna noticed Lexi appeared hesitant to discipline the kids. When asked about it privately, Lexi pushes back that it "isn't appropriate" for her in relation to the children. With the family in therapy, this could be addressed using a Venn diagram to explore how members define or view specific roles (teenager, parent, etc.) or behaviors (responsibility, discipline, etc.) that go with those roles. Here's an excerpt of that exercise in session:

Lexi:	"Well, Johanna described a good parent as someone preparing kids to be good adults. I guess that's something I can do, too, just maybe not in the same ways?"
Therapist:	"Wow, I hear a lot of depth in that answer. Tell me more about that."
L:	"Well, like I don't view myself as a stepparent, more as mom's partner. The kids call me Lexi, not a parent name like Mom or Dad."
T:	"And is it fair to say that not being Mom or Dad can feel a little lost, maybe? Like maybe you don't know what role you're supposed to have with the kids?" Lexi nods.
Johanna:	"I never knew you saw it that way."
T:	"That's exactly what this practice is for. It is so normal for us not to realize that there can be different views of what comes with different roles and ideas. Let's try another one, and this time, let's have Isaiah start. What does being a 'kid' mean to you? How are kids special and different from parents or grown-ups?"

Compassionate Contextualization

Here is a snippet addressing how Olivia can compassionately contextualize Lexi's emotions when Lexi tries to validate emotions at home:

Therapist:	"Olivia, Lexi just described how they can really see your point of view in your anger with your brother at that time, and also sees his perspective and understand his anger, too. What's different from how they said that now versus how they say it in the heat of the moment at home?"
Olivia:	"At home they say it all mad."
T:	"How can you tell they're mad?"
O:	"They rub their head, and go [exasperated sighing sound]."
T:	"And that means mad to you? [Olivia nods] I bet that doesn't feel good for you, huh? When else do adults make that sound, maybe when they aren't mad?"
O:	"Mama does that when she gets home every day, too."
T:	"Wow, and it doesn't mean she's mad then?"
O:	"No, just tired, I think." Johanna nods.
T:	"How might it make sense if Lexi is tired when you and your brother fight, not just mad?"
O:	"Maybe they're tired, too."
T:	"Tired, too? Does that mean you're tired when you fight with your brother, too?"
O:	"Sometimes."
T:	"Wow, great job noticing that about yourself! What else do you do when you get tired?" Olivia pauses, not answering. "May I ask others how they can tell when you're tired, and you give a thumbs up or down if they get it right?" She nods.

Disentangling

In family therapy, disentangling can also mean detriangulating. We talked about triangles back in Chapter 2, but triangulation is a specific type of relational dynamic between three people. Triangulation is the attempt to pull a third person into the problems of a dyad, usually with the goal of validating one person's perspective or to problem-solve an issue in the original pair. Detriangulating comes down to recognizing when an attempted triangulation is occurring and intentionally leaning away from the biases of that role. This is true as either the therapist and a family member. Remember, triangles are not automatically bad; triads can be nurturing, stable structures that provide emotional support through genuine seeking of understanding and endorsing congruent self-expression via open and safe communication, and improved self-esteem through authentic acceptance. A key attribute to create nurturing structures is emotional safety through emotional regulation, not suppression or reactivity. This is a key attribute of detriangulation, too. It is not by coincidence that both CRT and Satir highlight the triad between self, other, and context in fostering trust through mutual vulnerable authenticity and understanding.

How to notice you're being triangulated:

1. Are you being asked – directly or indirectly – to hold someone else's stress for them?
2. Does it seem obvious which of the other two people in the dyad is in the wrong?
3. Is someone avoiding conflict with someone else by turning to you instead?
4. Are resulting communication attempts or situational solutions short term (at best)?

How to disentangle a triangulation:

1. Identify nonjudgmentally to the person/people what is happening (*"It seems like I'm being emotionally pulled in to this issue between you and them"*).
2. Instead of fighting or shaming the person trying to pull you in (doing so would still an act of triangulation, just from the opposing perspective), offer compassionate contextualization for the act of triangulating a person, recognizing they may be reaching for validation of challenges or emotions around those challenges (*"It makes sense that you would turn to me if it feels scary or unhelpful to imagine confronting them directly"*).
3. Offer compassionate contextualization and conjecture of meaning-making and underlying emotions to each person's perspective in the triangle, whether they are present or not. (*"I wonder if they also are scared to talk to you directly about that."*)
4. Rotate attention on individual contributions to the negative feedback loop (the cycle that keeps the problem here) among all three people, not just the identified symptom bearer(s). This is rooted in taking accountability, not placing blame.

Positive Memory Restoration

Here is an example of a relational reflection between Johanna and Lexi about their different parenting styles, particularly when they were struggling with compassion:

T: "Jo, tell me about a time the past week when you felt really supported by Lexi as a parent."

J: "I honestly can't name one. It's been a while."

L: "Damn, that's harsh."

T: "Lexi, it sounds like that had some sting to it to hear Johanna say that. *When was a time you remember trying to offer support recently, maybe that went unnoticed?*"

L: "Well, she's been working late, right? So I have been trying to do more around the house, like having the kids fed and dishes done so she doesn't have to worry about it."

J: "But if you're making them microwave dinners, it's not exactly like that's really dinner or like they're really making dishes . . ."

T: "I can see where you're coming from, Jo. I can also hear the intent in Lexi's actions, here. They said they don't want you to worry about it. They want to take something off that endless mental list for you." Johanna nods. "*What is making it hard to see Lexi's attempt? Where is compassion hard right now?*"

J: "I mean, surely if they wanted me to not worry, they'd do better? Like Lex knows that's not the kind of dinners I want the kids to have."

T: "They know it's important to you for the kids to be well cared for, well fed." Johanna murmurs an agreement. "*How might it make sense if this is the best Lex has to offer right now, too?* Knowing it's important to you, they're giving what they can to support you and the kids."

J: "I mean, Lex has been busy, too. They work from home so many it's less obvious, but I get that sometimes our best just isn't what we want it to be."

T: "'Sometimes our best isn't what we want it to be.' What a heartfelt statement. It really speaks to the complexity of this situation. Lexi, *what do you hear Jo saying when she says she sees how busy you are, too?* That she sees that sometimes the situational best just isn't the ideal best?"

L: "That's what I need her to understand! I'm really trying to help. I know it isn't perfect, but neither is my cooking, and neither is she."

J: "I didn't say I was perfect!"

T: "Sounds like no one is saying that. Sounds like we are all humans trying to give the best we have right now. Jo, *tell me about a time when Lexi did prepare the kind of dinner you want the kids to have. How was life different then?*"

Temporary Agreements

Since this intervention is exemplified and referenced numerous times throughout this text, instead of giving a conversational example, let's list a few common examples of temporary agreements in family dynamics negotiations:

1. A minor's freedoms balanced with responsibilities
2. Sharing tactics between siblings
3. Activity participation, such as trying something new
4. Balancing individual versus family time and other scheduling details
5. Personal space or privacy

We will reiterate the intentional word choice here of *negotiating* and *managing*. People are more likely to "buy-in" or participate in a temporary agreement when they perceive they were a part of building it. Temporary agreements can be a space that we get to learn not only about what is important to different members of the family but why it is important, furthering that compassion.

Modality Comparison: Bowen's Multigenerational Family Therapy Model

As one of the earliest therapeutic modalities to come out of family systems theory, psychiatrist Murray Bowen designed Multigenerational Family Therapy model to explicitly look at the impact of systemic patterns on individual wellbeing. CRT takes cues from this model in the extensive and ongoing assessment as part of therapeutic interventions:

1. Collect history of the presenting problem
2. Find out what other mental and physical health treatment to system is receiving
3. Collect history of the nuclear family
4. Collect history of the extended family, such as parents' families of origin
5. Begin noting patterns, drawing attention to them conditionally
6. Identify patterns of blame given to family of origin for problematic behavior in the nuclear family
7. Create a genogram (a family tree of three or more generations reviewing family structures; relationship patterns; providing additional details such as ages of marriages, divorces, childbirths, deaths, and other significant life events and attributes such as illness, addiction, vocations, locations, spirituality, and other patterns potentially associated with the presenting problem)
8. Analyze the genogram, such as identifying cross-generational patterns

These questions frequently answer compassionate contextualization's core question, "How does it make sense I feel/think/act this way?" through the abundance of situational context provided. However, this and attentiveness to circularity may be the extent of similarities between the therapy models. Compared to Bowen's work, CRT places less emphasis on building higher self-differentiation as a therapeutic goal and does not simplify all systemic stress "anxiety," which could be considered an oversimplification and even minimizing to levels of distress tied to those stressors. That being said, the model does well highlighting the emotional states of others influencing oneself, which is part of compassionate contextualization. As CRT would say, others' thoughts, feelings, and behaviors affect our choices; they don't decide them. Exploring behaviors from nonjudgmental and curious language followed by presenting alternatives is a substantial piece of CRT family therapy.

Chapter 8

CRT with Children and Adolescents

According to existing research, self-compassion generally grows as people age. Of course, life experience and neurology impact this trajectory. For example, adolescents may have lower self-compassion due to burgeoning brain development, the belief in the personal fable, and imagined audience cognitive distortions common in youth. However, children can have a remarkable capacity for self-compassion and resilience, especially with the guidance of trusted adults. This chapter identifies contextual considerations for children and adolescents – including biological sex factors, distinct from the social construct of gender – based on their developmental stage and how to potentially adjust CRT interventions with these in mind and heart.

Contextualizing Child Development

People develop physically and cognitively consistently from birth into adulthood. Age and developmental stage impact their brains, sense of morality, and social priorities. These impact their behaviors. Psychoeducation and awareness about these can provide context and possible normalization (and therefore, compassion) for both the child and the adults in their lives. Compassion, validation, and normalization can help depersonalize attributes of the still-growing brain and body and the challenges that come with those ongoing changes.

Child Cognitive Development

Brain development can vary by sex of an individual early in life. Female brains are slightly smaller but tend to have larger limbic cortex (emotion management), hippocampus (memory), and frontal lobes (problem-solving) and more white matter (neural connections contributing to cognitive flexibility). Male brains are slightly larger with larger parietal cortex (spacial perception), hypothalamus (managing body sensations such as temperature,

DOI: 10.4324/9781003518730-10

hunger), and amygdala (stress regulation) and have more gray matter (muscle control and sensory perception). Based on early brain structure, children have a categorized, nominal understanding of the world. This results in frequent either/or language and linear comprehension ("If this, then that").

Impressively, meaning-making begins in infancy. It starts with language development – the idea a sound or symbol means an idea, thing, or action. From early life, children are sponges for information. They take in new words, cues, and behaviors and make sense of them based on previously known data. This is true of social skills, technical skills, and academic knowledge. In early to middle childhood, people begin to develop self-theory, marked by awareness of:

- Their independent existence
- Their ongoing existence (capacity to plan for the future)
- Their influence on their surroundings, including the environment and other people

Child Moral Development

In children, moral development is the shift from doing what is expected to doing what is right. It's following rules because it is congruent to your values, not because you might get in trouble if you don't. When younger, people tend to behave based on the desire to avoid punishment or receive praise. They are not intrinsically motivated by right or wrong. As children develop their sense of self, they also get a sense of the personal importance of adhering to cultural mores, or socialized rules such as waiting in line, using "please" and "thank you," and not being aggressive. Physical aggression as self-expression is common in younger children who may lack the language to express their needs or feelings in a situation. Moral development is associated with self-control, impulse control, and mirroring behaviors of the examples set to them (especially by adults and siblings).

Child Social Development

Since infancy, children lean on important adults in their lives to demonstrate emotional regulation and how to use them in communication. Attachment theory addresses this both as a matter of developing trust in adults to take care of them (secure attachment style) and demonstration of comfort and love. Secure attachment styles are associated with improved social competence, or the ability to form and maintain positive relationships with others.

Childhood peer relationships and sense of peer acceptance are also part of social competence. Lack of peer relationships can result in discomfort and self-doubt about initiating new friendships, hyperfocus on systematic exclusion ("cancel culture"), and increased helplessness and self-blame.

In addition to developing trust, childhood play and socialization encourages independent and cooperative problem-solving and creativity. As adults, we can ask and reflect, *"How are we encouraging creativity and curiosity and allowing mistakes and situational failures to be normalized as part of learning?"*

Contextualizing Adolescent Development

Adolescent development is most commonly thought of as puberty, or the physical shift to be able to reproduce. For girls, this typically takes 1–6 years, often begins around age 8–10, and is marked by breast development and menarche. For boys, puberty often takes 2–5 years; often begins around age 9–11; and is marked by growth in penis size, testicles, scrotal sac growth, and facial hair and change in voice. In both sexes, puberty is also associated with growth spurts, growth of pubic and underarm hair, and increased oil and sweat production. However, these are not the only changes and challenges of this age range and life stage.

Adolescent Cognitive Development

Brain development continues to around age 25, indicating adolescence carries well into one's theoretical adulthood. During this age, there are also significant changes in brain function:

1. Increased activity in the limbic system results in adolescents often being more emotionally reactive to negative stimuli than adults.
2. Increased dopamine activity results in increased maladaptive behaviors and risk-taking.

Both of these, combined with a burgeoning prefrontal cortex, means teenagers are aware of the potential risks in their behaviors but often minimize these if they do not see them as likely to happen to oneself or others.

Along with these changes, the horizontal control center (flow across brain hemispheres) enables executive control and verbal skills to overlap with emotional states. These are key to the development of formal operations thinking, including abstract thought:

- Juggling more than two variables in comprehension and decision-making
- Deductive reasoning, comprehension of logical consequences and logical inconsistency (attention to evidence, sensitivity to hypocrisy)

- Able to think more relativistically about self, others, and the world ("My norms are not everyone's")

Adolescent Moral Development

Adolescent morality relates to self-differentiation. As you may recall from Bowen's theory, self-differentiation is how a social system, such as a family, encourages a balance of relational intimacy and fostered independent identity. In adolescence, this means personally assessing laws, rules, and norms, particularly related to subjugated populations. To do this, adolescents will begin questioning and challenging previously taught values and identify the difference between social conventions from moral issues. The purpose of this is to begin designing one's own values.

While difficult for parents to cope with this deviation, it will be important not to personalize this as we normalize this process: It is not a failure of the parent for the child to have values different than those they were raised with. It is an important variation of fostering curiosity, as with childhood, to encourage people of all ages to reflect on why they hold the beliefs and values that they do. This is another version of compassionate contextualization in self-reflection tied to practicing internal and behavioral congruence.

Adolescent Social Development

Consistent with moral development, social development in adolescence is a self-synthesis that integrates past, present, and future versions of oneself into a comprehensive sense of identity. This includes one's values, beliefs, priorities, sense of purpose, interests, attitudes, self-expression, and the like. It is normal to experiment with one's identity/identifiers and self-expression throughout adolescence, such as appearance and clothing choices, gender and sexuality, hobbies and potential career aspirations, spirituality/religiosity, and systemic roles ("mom friend," "black sheep," "class clown," etc.). Adolescents begin personal meaning-making associated with identifiers connecting with macrosystems, such as what it means to belong to a specific faith, ethnic group, fan base, social group ("theater kid," "athlete," "nerd"), and the like. Some systemic roles will be placed on them, such as labels given by teachers, coaches, and parent figures. These can be positive ("helper"), demeaning ("problem child"), or restrictive, such as parentification ("man of the house").

This can be made challenging by the social emphasis on fitting into a social scheme. It is normal for adolescents to shift their attention from familial sense of belonging to peer sense of belonging. Additionally, this age is when romantic and sexual interests potentially begins, including desire for romantic relationship, increased physical arousal, and sense of sexual desire. However, high awareness of peer judgment and social implications of friendship and partner choices are still a factor.

A version of temporary agreements between adolescents and their mentors can be to give permission to not know and be "works in progress." This is not a statement of rejecting who they say they are ("It's just a phase"), but rather one of overlapping acceptance and openness to change as they learn more about themselves.

Limitations of CRT by Development Stage

This is a reiteration from Chapter 3. Psychoeducation can be beneficial only if the person is able to process the information and its abstract relevance. Children below 10–12 years old, the tail end of middle childhood, may lack the formal operational thinking that CRT leans into to differentiate one's experience from the experiences of others, put language to one's own perspective, and recognize one's bodily feelings and correlating emotions. Ability to understand self-compassion as a concept is also an essential cognitive and emotional baseline for CRT.

That being said, developmental stage and age are not a rigid line. As previously mentioned, early assessment includes listening for the client's emotional maturity, openness to differentiating emotional regulation from emotional suppression, and capacity for abstract thinking and ambiguity tolerance regardless of their age. Adults also have all of those considerations: What is their cognitive, moral, and social development status? In fact, there is a colloquial phrase that children with trauma history tend to present as mature for their age while simultaneously experiencing arrested development in other areas of life. This can be further accentuated when neurodivergence is present.

Contextualizing Adverse Childhood Experiences (ACEs)

Trauma in childhood impacts a person personally and socially, potentially for the remainder of their life. ACEs can result in neurological deficits and below-average pace of skill development. The following are commonly assessed ACEs:

1. Did you feel that you had enough to eat?
2. Did you have to wear dirty clothes?
3. Did you have inconsistent or unkempt housing, including being unhoused, in various foster homes, or living in a dirty home?
4. Did you feel that you had no one to protect or take care of you?

5. Did you lose a parent through divorce, abandonment, death, or other reason?
6. Did you live with anyone who was depressed, mentally ill, or attempted or completed suicide?
7. Did you live with anyone who had a problem with drinking or using drugs, including prescription drugs?
8. Did you live with anyone who went to jail or prison?
9. Did your parents or adults in your home ever physically injure or threaten to harm each other?
10. Did your parents or adults in your home ever physically injure or threaten to harm other children in the home?
11. Did a parent or adult in your home ever physically injure or threaten to harm you in any way?
12. Did a parent or adult in your home ever swear at you, insult you, or put you down?
13. Did you feel that no one in your family loved you or thought you were special?
14. Did you experience unwanted sexual contact (such as fondling or oral/anal/vaginal intercourse/penetration)?

Though not frequently asked about, chronic illness of a person or a loved one in the home, another form of trauma contributing to parentification or victimization, can also contribute to cognitive and/or social delay.

Per CRT, ACEs are context; they let us know what possible stressors a child's life has included so far. Current ACEs can also be contraindications for therapy as we prioritize their physical and emotional safety. ACEs can also cue us into someone's capacity for compassion, in minors and/or adults. Children who experience more ACEs are more likely to:

o experience poor physical health, chronic disease, and premature mortality;
o exhibit violent, reactive aggressive, or criminal behavior later in life;
o display psychopathic behavior and affect such as manipulation, dishonest charm, callousness, and unemotionality;
o increase likelihood of substance abuse;
o decrease in positive affect;
o increase in negative affect, emotional dysregulation, and self-regulation deficits;
o show feelings like abandonment, insecurity, and solitude, affecting their self-esteem and the ability to socialize with others decreased altruistic attitudes; and

o have insecure attachment styles (anxious, avoidant, detached), including in adulthood. This is because children develop beliefs and behavior patterns based on the relationship they have with their primary caregiver.

Emotional abuse and family dysfunction, specifically, are risk factors for pedophilia, exhibitionism, rape, or multiple paraphilias, with emotional abuse contributing more significantly than family dysfunction.

Stress, such as from ACEs, greatly impacts early brain development. It restricts development in executive functioning (associated self-control, problem-solving, decision-making, planning, organization, and attention and time management) and memory. These must also be taken into consideration in both assessment and intervention methods in CRT.

Additional Assessment Considerations with Minors

If a client system includes a child, it is essential to include them in the assessment process. While it may require more patience and some creativity than collecting data solely from an adult, children offer invaluable insight to a system's functionality and built-in meaning-making. That is to say, parents may not realize what message is being received by their behaviors and words, and there's no better place than therapy to explore that. When working with minors, there are a few other variables to consider from the very beginning of the therapeutic process:

• When doing assessment questions with children, be mindful that they are susceptible to memory suggestion. When asking for their version of events, be aware of this filter, especially if the adults are present. Listen for adult-like language or skewed perspectives on people or issues they know little about. This is especially true of potentially legally mandated reportable situations, such as current ACEs. In such times, it will be important to reiterate confidentiality and safety priorities in child-comprehensive language.
• Be very attentive to nonverbals. While also true of adults, there is a reason the phrase, "Actions speak louder than words" is so popular. Sometimes people's emotions or thoughts are more congruent to their behaviors than their speech. For example, it can be very telling if you ask a child a question and they look to a parent to answer rather than answer for themselves.
• Be intentional to include children in the treatment planning and goals. What are highs and lows of their relationships (joyful and difficult memories)? How will they know when things are better – how might they or their loved ones act differently at that time?

- Lastly, it is the professional's responsibility to know your jurisdiction's legal requirements. This includes mandated reporting, guardian involvement in therapy, age of mental health treatment consent, and definitions of gender-affirming care and its legality with minors, to name a few. Frequently check the laws of your state, providence, and/or country to stay up-to-date.

Alternative Structure CRT Interventions

As is often the case, change in children and adolescents is rooted in change in the system, particularly the adults they spend the most time with. Live-in adults, in particular, contribute to skill development in six ways:

1. How they place value on the skill as important.
2. How they emphasize the benefit of the skill as helpful.
3. How they make materials associated with the skill available at home.
4. How they spend time with children demonstrating the skill *and* helping the child do the skill.
5. Demonstrating when and how to use the skill.
6. Frequency and quality of verbal interaction between parent and child.

Therefore, several interventions, even those focused on children, incorporate family members. CRT's interventions can be shifted to be creative and experiential/"gamified" to appeal with children without leaning heavily on insight.

Psychoeducation

Remember, the purpose of psychoeducation in CRT is to normalize and validate experiences. With children and adolescents in particular, it is important to go slow and in small increments to avoid overwhelming anyone. After giving a few sentences of information, therapists can request nonverbal feedback of applicability (*"On a scale of thumbs up to thumbs down, how true does this information seem to you and your life? Or, shrug for if you don't understand the question."*).

As usual, psychoeducation can also be used in compassionate contextualization from an adult toward a child (*"I can see why that was so hard!"*). With adolescents, a concern is frequently feeling misunderstood, so it can be helpful to convey understanding or seeking understanding from curiosity, not criticism or correction (*"I don't understand, but I want to. I know it makes sense to her with her perspective and life experience."*). Family camaraderie – the sense that our family is on the same team – is a significant contextual attribute that perpetuates emotional safety. It affirms that curiosity is a good thing, not a threat to family connection or identity.

Intentional Language

Three attributes of CRT's intentional language that particularly resonate with children are metaphors, parts, and friend-like language. These can be talked about; drawn; or roleplayed through storytelling or with toys, stuffed animals, or pillows and weighted blankets.

- *Metaphors* work well when it might be hard to name or describe emotions or how you need compassion. It may be easier to consider how a golden retriever gives and receives compassion without questioning their worthiness of it.
- *Parts language* overlaps with "both/and" language, such as how a parent can be both a source of fear and love. Referencing movies like Disney/Pixar's *Inside Out* can be a culturally familiar example children can use to make sense of their own "internal family" of parts and how they interact with one another. The therapist can tie in these known references by asking, *"How does it make sense a part of you feels so angry?"*
- *Friend-like language* offers a pseudo-externalization option for how children talk about compassion: *"If you had a friend going through something like this, how would you comfort them?"* or, *"How would you hope a friend would show their love and support to you right now?"* There are also versions for parent-like language: *"How would you hope your parent would show . . ."*

Children, being the sponges they are and relatively easy to influence, are often eager to practice new skills and language. While the language might be introduced with the child, including parental figures in on these can be helpful so they can use the language or tool at home, too.

Compassionate Contextualization

For individuals who learn with tactile skill building, there is an experiential version of compassionate contextualization that includes moving in a baseball diamond-shaped motion while offering self-compassion (see Figure 8.1).

- *Home base* – place your hand on your chest, and take a deep, slow inhale through your nose to see the hand rise, and slowly exhale through your mouth. Ask yourself, "What am I feeling/thinking/doing that is sitting unwell with me?"

- *First base* – pause to feel your heartbeat in your palm, and take another slow breath in and out. Ask yourself, "How does it make sense I feel/think/did that?"
- *Second base* – pat or rub a small circle on your chest over your heart, taking another slow breath in and out. State to yourself, "It is understandable you feel/think/behaved this way. It makes sense, all things considered." If there is an opposing critical voice, such as someone saying, "You should know better!" or "How could you not know that?" you can answer that with, "When would you have learned that?" or, "Even if I know, how does it make sense I didn't think if it at that moment?"
- *Third base* – take another slow inhale and exhale. Ask yourself, "What do I need right now?" This could include physical sensations such as being tired, hungry or thirsty, temperature dysregulation, discomfort in your clothes, or wanting to cry. Offer to yourself when you will be able to address this as soon as possible, immediately if this is an option.
- *Home run* – taking another deep breath, offer a statement of gratitude to yourself. For example, "Thank you for pausing to notice my needs. I have value, and so do they. We will continue to learn to accept our humanness together," or something similar.

This mindfulness practice serves to meld physical movement and self-soothing (physical touch, slowed breathing, etc.).

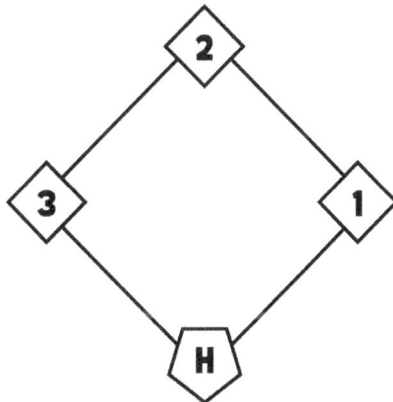

Figure 8.1 Compassionate Contextualization Diamond

Disentangling

Continuing the theme of using visual variations of CRT interventions, here are a few focuses in disentangling:

- Disentangling differences in meaning-making while seeking overlap between people's perspectives can be created as a Venn diagram. Children often benefit from visual aids to hold their attention and give space for them to participate, such as writing answers.
- To disentangle linear assumptions, we can draw a road for imagery of possible *"forks in the road"* of possibilities, including fears and hopes, tied to the questions of, *"What else could be true?"* or, *"What else could happen?"* and furthering the metaphor with questions such as, *"How does it feel to not know which road we're on when we take it?"* This option, in particular, can be used to encourage creativity and problem-solving scenarios for children's cognitive development and adolescent autonomy development.

Particularly with adolescents, it can be helpful to explore what "I don't know" means to someone, as it can communicate many different ideas (see Figure 8.2).

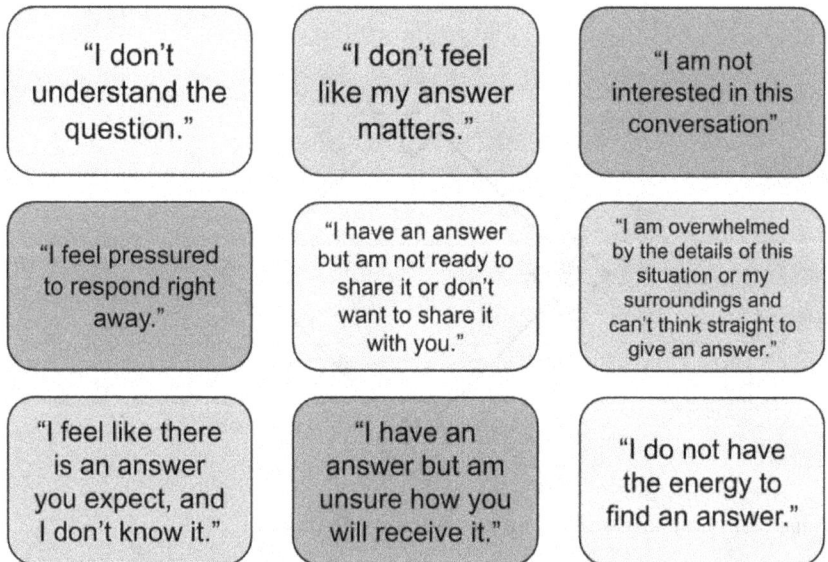

Figure 8.2 Clarifying "I Don't Know"

As always, it is also important to clarify the purpose of communication:

1. Wanting to share/vent, validation response only
2. Seeking sympathy, comfort, celebration
3. Seeking input or advice

(If multiple, go in this order.)

Positive Restorations

Across all ages and developmental levels, positive restorations focuses on how compassion can be or has been present and enjoyable aspects of a relationship are not overlooked. One method to practice this – and retain a visual reminder of felt love and progress toward compassion and self-compassion – is to draw a positive memory: "Draw a picture for me of a time you felt connected, understood, appreciated, loved, and grateful for?" These are the same relational reflection questions as we ask adults, and we can do the same for compassionate preparation questions, too.

Temporary Agreements

With adolescents, temporary agreement can simply be permission for identities to be temporary or have ongoing exploration. Since minors are sensitive to consistency, having a written contract, identifying each person's responsibilities and the reward for completion, can be helpful to set clear expectations. For some people, having a visual guide for kids to note the passing time between when an agreement is made and when it ends can also be a useful method to eliminate ambiguity where possible. In either case, there is space for compassion in the difficulty of transitions, change, and new structures, offering validation to one another.

One of the first temporary agreements we make with kids and adolescents, is to HALT and not attempt emotionally intense conversations when *Hungry*, *Angry*, *Lonely*, or *Tired*. However, the second part of the agreement is to pick a time, such as 30 minutes later, to come back to the conversation.

Modality Comparison: Internal Family Systems Therapy

Internal Family Systems Therapy (IFS) began with a family therapist noticing a client naturally using parts language: "A part of me feels one way, but another wants something completely different." Dick Schwartz, the theory's originator, saw peoples' parts tended to fall into two categories: exiled parts that carried deep, often hurtful, beliefs about oneself rooted in rejection and unworthiness, and protector parts that worked hard to either proactively avoid that belief being reiterated (managers) or responded swiftly when a situation made that belief seem true (firefighters). These parts fell into interaction cycles and patterns, both within an individual and between members of a system, such as a family. Parts are aspects of oneself, led by a Core Self, seeking a sense of security and functionality within oneself and one's relationships.

CRT uses parts language but is not specific to the roles of managers, firefighters, and exiles. While we might not use the language of Core Self to describe the internal sense of peace and self-assuredness within ourselves, we do endorse the attributes IFS gives to this aspect of oneself: calm, creative, curious, connected, confident, courageous, clarity, and *compassionate*. We also agree with the notion of no parts being bad, and those that are outspoken simply seek to be heard and loved.

As mentioned earlier, parts language can work well with children because it embraces their innate creativity and curiosity. We can use imagery, artistic expression, and modified externalization to recognize that parts of us can identify individual attachment wounds in need of love and reassurance in addition to sources of joy that we can share in with loved ones.

Chapter 9

Compassionate Boundaries

When you think of boundaries, what do you think of? Some people think of a physical boundary, like a fence outlining a property edge. Some people think of difficult memories when "no" was not respected and a relational boundary was crossed. Both of these are types of boundaries; this chapter specifically focuses on the latter.

We introduced boundaries as a family systems theory concept back in Chapter 2. To briefly review, the purpose of boundaries is to establish relational and/or personal safety by setting relationship-appropriate limits. They aim to minimize under- and over-functioning and maximize optimal functioning. This allows the individuals in the relationship to feel more secure in their role with the other person(s).

We frequently tell clients that boundaries are about managing yourself, not about controlling someone else. They are, by themselves, an act of compassion toward oneself and the hope for the future of that relationship. The boundary will, of course, influence other people, who may push back simply because it is new and unknown. Contextually, the unknown can be scary, threatening, and disconnecting! It makes sense.

The purpose of compassionate boundaries is to convey a boundary not as a threat but actually a constructive tool to let the relationship find its best form. That being said, the best form may vary situationally. The practice of setting, following through with consistency, and continuing to take care of that relationship primes the safety for those fluctuations.

How Boundaries Improve Relationships

Conversations about boundaries are becoming more commonplace. What boundaries look like, expectations around them, and expressing versus assuming have become more frequent topics of conversation. Research tells us that setting and maintaining boundaries in life and relationships are fundamental for emotional wellbeing. It is a way to establish appropriate emotional differentiation, balancing influence and independence. Learning

DOI: 10.4324/9781003518730-11

how to create and keep healthy, nonrigid boundaries is a form of self-love and reclamation. Doing so can improve quality and satisfaction in relationships as everyone learns the roles and responsibilities together.

For example, consider when parents become empty-nesters. Their kids move away, and suddenly, the way they have parented so far – being physically present to oversee the child's development – is no longer an option. As a college student, my friend's mother would come to her dorm every weekend. While visiting, she did her adult daughter's laundry, housekeeping, took her shopping, and bought her take-out food instead of going to the cafeteria. My friend told me it bothered her, and she felt like her mom was "overstepping." But she didn't want to disappoint her mom or hurt her feelings, so she let her mom continue to be this version of "mom." No one knew how that role needed to adjust to accommodate the change in life stage, nor how to communicate that.

Role clarification is the key reason boundaries improve relationships. It articulates clear expectations of how each person can relate to the other and understand what the other needs, personified by the behaviors.

Steps to Set Compassion-Based Boundaries

Setting compassionate boundaries is a balance of directness and gentleness – remember, direct does not have to mean confrontational or harsh. The steps to do this are:

1. State the desired boundary or interaction dynamic.
2. If the boundary is pushed/crossed, state your intended response to it happening again.
3. As needed, follow through the response.
4. Self-soothe.

As we begin this conversation, remind yourself it is never too late to set a needed boundary. It does not have to be that you failed to set one earlier; boundaries can change as life circumstances do, like the example with my college friend. Changes in boundaries are a normal experience coinciding with stage of life transitions, and they are also acceptable even as our physical, emotional, and relational needs change over time. Let's go over the details of each of these steps.

State the desired boundary or interaction dynamic.

From the beginning, it is important to state that clients get to decide for themselves what boundaries feel acceptable and hoped for in their relationships, including with the therapist. It is not for the therapist to determine. When setting a boundary, two features are helpful:

1A. Identify the potential mutual benefit.
1B. Identify the emotions impacting the boundary (both as the setter and recipient).

Identifying the mutual benefit emphasizes the intention of the boundary to be relationship building, not harming. For example, "I want both of us to feel safe to express when something the other says is uncomfortable."

Identifying the emotions of the situation highlights the speaker's humanness – this is not a heartless proclamation, unphased by the emotions of the recipient. The frustration, grief, disappointment, fear, or guilt surrounding setting the boundaries, or having someone set them with us, is an important part to process. You don't have to pretend this is easy! It is human to say, "I know this isn't easy to hear, and it isn't easy to say, either," or, "I know I previously seemed fine with it, and after thinking on it, I realized I'm not. I feel bad for having given the wrong impression." Similarly, it is fair to give space for the recipient to share their feelings, too.

Sometimes, step one is all that's needed. People can hear your desired boundary and respect it. However, this is not always the case.

If the boundary is pushed/crossed, state your intended response to it happening again.

As with step 1, this includes two features:

2A. Identify your next response action
2B. Identify the next initiation of contact along with a statement of love

It is important to emphasize that this process is a consequence, not a punishment. This is the practice of overt, preemptive communication so the person receiving the boundary is not left guessing what will happen next.

Setting a boundary does not have to be severe. The most extreme example is a total cut-off of communication, or an end of the relationship. However, there are more temporary options that allow the relationship to continue overall:

o Ending the current conversation or interaction
o Ending a current visit, leaving a physical space
o Canceling a future plan or no longer volunteering your time for certain events

Identifying the next initiation of contact serves two purposes. Primarily, it reiterates the importance of the ongoing relationship. It offers an opportunity to demonstrate to the recipient that you follow through on all parts of the boundary, including reconnection (for you both!). If the future of the relationship does not influence you (such as a cat-caller or stranger), it is not necessary to speak of future contact and is up to the individual if they feel emotionally or physically safe to state why they are ending the interaction, such as walking away or silently refusing to engage with the person(s).

Sometimes, the recipient of the boundary may attempt to negotiate both the boundary and next contact. Different people have different feelings about this, frequently dependent on previous experiences with these situations, people, and settings (compassionate contextualization). It is up to the individual how to respond to attempts to do so. Approaching this with compassion both for the setter and recipient, acknowledging nonjudgmentally why this might be a difficult experience, is also why reiteration of love is so important.

As needed, follow-through the response.

Setting and holding boundaries are challenging as independent steps; we can compassionately contextualize this, as well. This follow through shows the recipient that the setter is true to their word, including the potential next contact plans.

Nonetheless, the recipient may push back. That's part of the process as they attempt to reclaim a sense of control in the situation/relationship, or to regain previously held power dynamics. They may make their own statements of impending cut-off, maybe calling these boundaries of their own in response to the first. That's okay; as not fun as it is, they are allowed to do that. People might not respond well, and that is their responsibility to emotionally process, not yours. Frequently, the setter following through on the next initiation of contact eases this slightly. Consistency will be the most securing factor as the relational shift occurs.

Another common response can be a claim to not know the setter would follow through, possibly based on previous experience or their own assumptions. In such times, it is fair to compassionately acknowledge the difference between ignorance (not knowing), indifference (not caring), and inconsideration ("I know this matters to you, but I don't want to change") by the boundary crosser. However, we must not make assumptions of our own of which is the case.

If a boundary is pushed back on, based on the boundary, it can be appropriate to either reiterate the emotional challenges of the boundary and the next planned contact, or remain silent if that is necessary to protect the boundary and yourself.

Self-soothe

Apply the compassionate contextualization diamond: Check in with yourself – how does it make sense that setting and holding boundaries is hard? Maybe there is a history of people-pleasing. Maybe the person on the receiving end has a history of misplacing their emotions onto other people, such as yourself, and that's uncomfortable. Discomfort, like any emotion, has a subjectively logical source.

Next, think about how you can show up for yourself throughout this process. Do you need space or closeness with another trusted loved one? A way to access the emotions behind the act of setting boundaries? Someone supportive to talk to about the experience in the moment? Physical movement to release the emotion, such as a walk, stretching, dance, or strength-training exercises? Ultimately, self-soothing is compassion for why boundaries feel challenging to set, hold, and receive. Nonjudgmentally reflecting in this allows the headspace to look at the boundary's success or futility to achieve the desired relational roles and rules.

Boundaries are an example of a temporary agreement. We try something, see how it works, and change as needed, communicating throughout. If a cut-off happens, it can be short term. Ask yourself:

- How would I know when/if I was ready to reengage or accept someone else's reinitiation? What would be different in how I think, act, or feel then compared to now?
- Am I open to other perspectives, even those I disagree with?
- Am I practicing self-soothing outside of therapy?
- Do my emotions still quickly overwhelm me?

Asking these types of questions may convey to yourself how ready you are to engage with the other person.

Notice none of these steps include a requirement of explanation for the boundary. It is not required, and often can feel counterproductive as the recipient may twist or use logical fallacies to reject those explanations and therefore the need for the boundary. Instead, if asked, "Why?," we can reference back to the potential mutual benefit and ongoing love for the person.

Coping with Relational Fallout

Everyone handles boundaries, particularly changes in boundaries, differently. The CRT approach includes increasing capacity and compassion for self and others surrounding the challenges of boundary work. When exploring client boundaries, even compassionately, there are pieces the therapist will want to address with clients:

- The person you set boundaries with might interact with you differently after, such as being more distant than before. This may be a temporary adjustment, or long term, perhaps even as part of the desired outcome. This is a common point of uncertainty as the relationship may feel insecure during the transition.
- Topics that may have been assumed "acceptable" before may not be anymore. Again, this may be by design (intentionally part of the new boundary) or a byproduct of the boundary taken to an extreme. For example, a person may decide to no longer accept invitations to religious gatherings (attend church/mass, mosque, temple, etc.), and their family may not know how to talk about faith with them at all anymore, now that the previously assumed aligned religion-affiliated values no longer apply.
- There may be a shift in power dynamics. Often, the hope is for more egalitarian sense of relational safety and/or role clarification, particularly if a hierarchy is maintained.

With any of these, it is beneficial to offer compassionate contextualization and experience-based validation to self, others, and situation. You can explore these in session or have the person(s) practice these at home individually or together.

Intergenerational and Cultural Boundary Considerations

Based on social and personal experiences, different generations often have unique perspectives on what ideal, healthy boundaries look like and why they are necessary. Intergenerational boundaries can be especially challenging to facilitate based on competing expectations of what is normal or healthy. Generations who assume disagreement is synonymous to disrespect have a harder time accepting boundaries, particularly from their children. Individuals raised to believe relational restrictions are innately disloyal also struggle with boundaries. There are many factors:

- Taught definition and meaning-making of boundaries
- Reinforced people-pleasing in upbringing
- Taught prioritization between systems and self
- Given or felt pressure or obligation (at an extreme, lack of consent)
- Sense of entitlement (the right to influence)

- Sense of self-worth
- Taught adaptability

These attributes are not exclusive to generational differences; similar perspectives can be held based on cultural values.

Cultural values also greatly impact perceptions of boundaries. When looking at collectivist approaches versus individualistic approaches, which intensely value autonomy and personal achievement, we can see how desired boundaries could look different. In some, enmeshment is the norm. The assumption is that family is entitled to intimately know about the lives of loved ones because self-regulation and personal wellbeing is dependent on that emotional overlap. This is not innately destructive but can be if held strictly. Boundaries can be received as not only personal rejection but a rejection of cultural identity.

Rigid individuality can also be destructive. These people may be quick to cut relationships off on the grounds of prioritizing personal wellbeing. This can be the risky extreme version of differentiation, which rejects the relational reality that people are inevitably influenced, even inversely, by their upbringing. Rigid individuality of the boundary-setter can actually damage role clarification intentions in boundaries.

Of course, these are two ends of a spectrum across macrosystems, exosystems, and microsystems. This can be further complicated by the growing normality of multicultural systems, such as mixed-race marriages, immigrant families, and workplaces that span multiple communities and countries.

Ultimately, based on this complexity, it is common for people to have personal definitions of preferred boundaries, developed over personal life experiences and meaning-making of boundaries.

In a therapy context, prepare for there to be different perceptions and assumptions of boundaries as a practice (meaning-making). These will need to be overtly explored, such as asking, *"What do you believe healthy boundaries look like?"* or *"Tell me about a time when you felt respected and loved even when disagreed with."*

Boundaries, Hierarchy, and Power

Across both generational and cultural influences, there is a theme of maintaining hierarchy. Hierarchy is the ranking of power and responsibility, or role clarity. In older generations and collectivistic cultures, social hierarchy is well defined and ingrained. This can result in a greater perceived authoritarian leadership with little to no permission to question or explore system rules and expectations; even asking about such things directly can be perceived as challenging them. In established hierarchies, who or what has the power to set those rules also impacts where and when one sets boundaries. In other systems, power reinforced by hierarchy is less affixed or observable. Systems that value democratic or egalitarian division of leadership may approach rules, roles, and boundaries as more negotiable and changeable over time.

Neither of these are inherently correct. With younger children, a well-established hierarchy is an essential attribute to teaching social mores, life skills, and critical thinking skills. This is developmentally reasonable; parents place rules that a child's brain development may not comprehend:

- "If you go outside in the snow, wear your boots."
- "Come tell me if you accidentally break something; don't keep it to yourself."
- "Put your finished homework back in your bag when you're done so you don't forget it in the morning."

Since parents are viewed as responsible for their child(ren)'s wellbeing, it makes sense that they might be more structured in the rules and roles distinguishing adult and child to avoid legal consequence. From an early age, parents can use boundaries as a disciplinary phrasing of cause and effect. As I frequently remind my clients who are parents, the Latin origin of "discipline" means both "to learn" and "to teach."

As children grow and develop into their own personalities and perspectives, the former hierarchy may no longer fit. In our earlier example of empty-nesters, the tasks associated with the role of a parent change once the young adult leaves the home. There may even come a time in life when the adult child may intercede to be hierarchically over their parents in some ways as caretakers when elderhood brings physical or mental limits.

When setting and holding boundaries impacting hierarchy structures, it can be helpful to reiterate maintained role titles ("You're still Mom") and capabilities related to autonomy and power ("You can still be the one to coach me through the yardwork"). It is significant in CRT to acknowledge the advantage of hierarchies situationally, along with the necessity of their transition over time: *"Knowing about the world this person grew up in, the values they were taught, how does it make sense that they have the view of boundaries that they do? That they parented the way they did? That your child is setting this limit now?"*

Modality Comparison: Structural Family Therapy

In both CRT and structural family therapy, there is emphasis on role clarity and the setting of positive examples by parental or significant adult figures to other system members, such as children or extended family members. However, the two models approach this quite differently. Structural emphasizes creating appropriate hierarchy between familial generations or leadership positions to clarify decision-making dynamics between individuals. CRT leans into role clarification as a trust-building boundary not to affirm power differences across generations but to decrease role or expectation ambiguity. With decreased ambiguity, we see increased felt relational and autonomous safety and improved demonstration of internal and behavioral coping methods. Per recent research, role clarity and structure-based systemic interventions have been shown to decrease cognitive and behavioral problems in adolescents, create higher family cohesion, improve relational satisfaction, and implementation of parental practices and perceived efficacy as a parent.

Structural family therapy introduced a tool/intervention called the family map that could also be helpful in CRT. Completed by each member of the family, this can be either a drawn graphic or experiential activity called family sculpting, positioning people's posture and location around a room. It focuses on how a family is organized, portraying perceived closeness, distance, or exclusion and each person's "size" of influence in the family. Having each person complete this aids to wordlessly provide different perceptions, including children. Figure 9.1 is an example of how this could look with Johanna's nuclear family, per Olivia's view.

As people describe their maps, therapists can fold in emotional conjecture (*"I see some teariness from Mom; I wonder if this is really impacting her to see how Liv sees the family"*), compassionate contextualization (*"How does it make sense that Olivia views Mom as the*

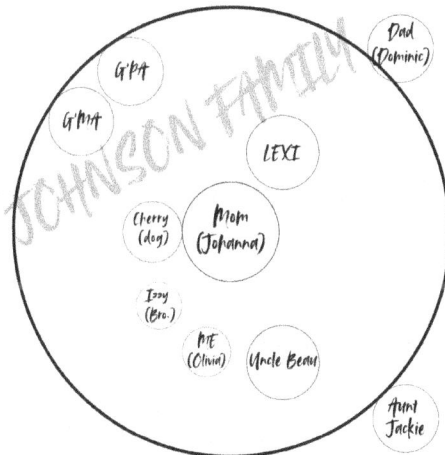

Figure 9.1 Case Example Structural Map

center of the family circle, or center of family focus?"), or disentangling meaning-making (*"If you were to view this from your child's perspective, what significance could there be to Mom and Lexi being close but their circles not quite touching?"*). This activity does more than provide insight; it provides space to acknowledge the emotions that underlie insight – loneliness, hurt, sadness, pain – and a place to practice comfort and compassion in response. We learn about others' perceptions of our boundaries, and we use temporary agreements to explore how we can meet the needs of both the boundary setter and the person seeking connection and comfort, too.

Case Example

Let's come back to Johanna and her family once more. In past sessions, we've heard about Dominic, Johanna's former spouse and Olivia and Isaiah's father. In an earlier session with the children present, Johanna indicated that she struggles in her communications with Dominic but indicated she wanted to talk about this without the children present.

This, by itself, is an excellent boundary to set in therapy. In their family structure, based on the children's age and ongoing relationship with their father, Johanna intentionally does not want to disclose challenges between her and Dominic in front of them. Therefore, a session was scheduled with her and Lexi to explore that relationship. This is an excerpt of the next session; the interventions are italicized where used:

Therapist:	"So, last time you were here, you signaled you didn't want to talk about the communication issues with Dominic in front of the children, which is fair. What are the thoughts or emotions that come with talking about him?"
Johanna:	"Honestly, overwhelm and immediate exhaustion. Even after three years, Dom still texts me these comments, like calling me names or insulting Lexi . . ."
Lexi:	"I really don't care. He's the bitch for being so petty. Last week, right before we saw you, Jo texted asking if he could take them on our anniversary weekend. He replied shaming her for 'trying to get rid of them for her own pleasures,' and refused because it's not his weekend."
J:	"He doesn't even have plans! He's just being difficult out of spite."

T: "Wow! Even hearing you describe this, I can feel the overwhelm and exhaustion from you. It makes so much sense that you would feel that way with those interactions. Lexi, what is it like for you to see your wife feel so overwhelmed and exhausted related to the kids' father?" *[compassionate contextualization, circular questioning]*

L: "I mean, it pisses me off. She shouldn't have to deal with him being so immature."

T: "Mmm, I can see that. I do want to follow up on Johanna's assumption that he is acting solely out of spite. I want to catch that because we don't know, right? We can strongly suspect, but we don't know. And if we treat that assumption like it's fact, it might affect how we respond instead of actually getting to address the issue, right?" *[identifying assumption of intent]*

J: "That's fair."

T: "With that in mind, what would you each say is the actual issue?"

J: "How he talks to me. I tried to set a boundary back when we were just separated to only talk about the kids, because back then he would call me and leave messages just yelling at me and blaming me for everything."

T: "I imagine that was really hurtful; I bet that stung." *[emotion conjecture]* "Jo, tell me more about the boundary you tried to set earlier. How did you reinforce it when he pushed it?"

J: "If I'm honest, I didn't. I just asked him not to talk to me like that and that we only talk about the kids. I would just not respond when he would try something else. Lexi started just deleting the messages from him without me hearing or reading them first."

T: "That sounds like a held boundary to me! Maybe the cause-and-effect wasn't stated, but you responded with silence, aiming to discourage him from continuing that behavior." *[exception- based strength highlighting]*

J: "That's true."

T: "How do you wish he would interact with you instead?" *[identify desired situation]*

J: "I wish we only texted like once a week about whatever is going on with the kids that week."

T:	"How do you believe that would be beneficial to you, Lexi, maybe even Dom?"
J:	"I mean, I don't want him stewing in negativity, either. I just want to focus on what matters - the kids."
T:	"What would it be like to send a message to him stating that, and trying a follow-through, just for the next week or so?" *[temporary agreement]*
J:	"Terrifying but probably worth it."
T:	"Let's take a breath and pause here. How does it make sense it can be both terrifying and worth it? Where are you feeling that terror inside you?" *[and language compassionate contextualization with mindfulness]*

From here, the session would explore the crafting of the message to send, what follow-through Johanna would be comfortable to try, and what self-soothing looks like for her, offering compassionate contextualization throughout.

Steps to Set & Hold Compassionate Boundaries:

State the desired interaction dynamic:
- Make the request
- Identify potential mutual benefit
- Identify emotions impacting the boundary

Example:
"Mom, please don't call me on Sundays. I want us both to have our personal time honored so we can relax."

If pushed/crossed, state the intended response if it happens again:
- Identify next action in an "if, then" statement
- If appropriate, identify next point of contact, including offering of love

Example:
"If you call me again on Sunday, I won't answer, but I'll call you on Tuesday after work. I love you and will talk to you then."

Follow through as necessary:
- Prepare for push-back, this is a normal response to new boundaries
- Either reiterate the current boundary, offer another, or stay silent, depending on the situation

Example:
"If you insist on calling me Sundays, we won't talk Tuesday, either, because I feel very disrespected right now."

Self-soothe:
- How do your current emotions make sense about how this boundary is being received?
- Self-validate – This is not an easy process!
- What does my body need right now? Rest? Movement? Food?
- What does my heart need right now? Space for further personal reflection? Space to cry? A friend to talk to?

Repeat as needed.

What are Boundaries?
- Boundaries are the rules that convey relationship dynamics. They create personal and relational safety
- Setting compassionate boundaries is a balance of directness and gentleness - direct does not have to mean confrontational/harsh
- Boundaries are not a threat or telling someone else what they can do; it is a management of your behavior, not theirs
- It is never too late to set a needed boundary!

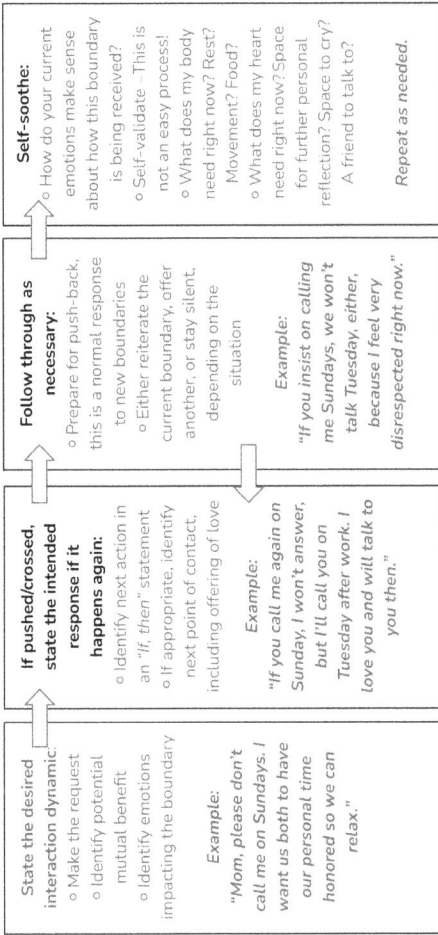

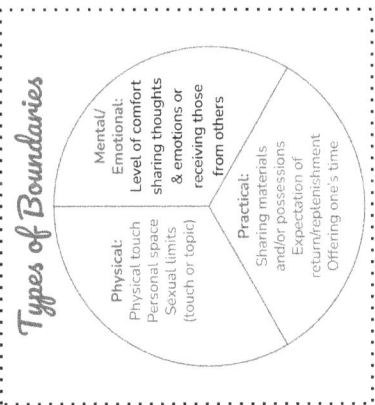

Examples of Boundaries (other than cut-off)
- Leaving a room/space, ending a phone call
- Ending a game when someone cheats
- Not sharing treasured belongings
- Requesting to be asked before a hug
- Not responding to a cat-caller
- Not hosting an event
- Keeping time to yourself
- Unfollowing someone on social media
- Only meeting someone in public or for a limited time
- Choosing not to give information (privacy ≠ secrecy)

Types of Boundaries

Mental/ Emotional: Level of comfort sharing thoughts & emotions or receiving those from others

Physical: Physical touch Personal space Sexual limits (touch or topic)

Practical: Sharing materials and/or possessions Expectation of return/replenishment Offering one's time

Figure 9.2 Compassionate Boundaries Guide & Infographic

Part III

Romantic Relationship Therapy Application

Chapter 10

Compassionate Relational Romantic Therapy

In the minimal existing research about it, compassion has consistently demonstrated itself to be beneficial to romantic relationships, and growth in self-compassion positively correlates with growth in romantic relationship satisfaction and positive regard. In Part 3 of this text, we will utilize CRT with romantic relationships. We will discuss what this looks like in different romantically relational contexts and use case studies to demonstrate CRT concepts, highlighting specific relational dynamics. This includes some specific relationship challenges and dynamics, such as infidelity and navigating ethical nonmonogamy, and we will explore what CRT brings to the table in these situations.

Romantic Relationship Contexts to Consider

As mentioned in Chapter 2 and as systematic thinkers, we are always considering the different contexts impacting the client in front of us:

• Family values and normalized thoughts and behaviors
• Macro- and microsystemic influences
• How they learned to cope and connect (or disconnect) when growing up, etc.

However, in romantic partnership therapy, there's even more information in the space for us to process and work with. Oftentimes in relational work, we're bringing together two or more families of influence:

• Meaning-making of individual and shared life events (both past and present)
• Different values and belief systems
• Co-occurring stage of life obligations

DOI: 10.4324/9781003518730-13

Put another way, when we work with two or more individuals, we are also working with their relationships as if they are an additional member of the client system. While true in families, this can be particularly complicated in romantic partnerships as we bring together more contextual factors along the way:

- Romantic relationship histories (previous relationships)
- Romantic relationship history (their relationship)
- Relationship strengths and weaknesses; high points and low points of the current relationship

That being recognized, it makes sense that the assessment continues throughout the therapy process with romantic relationships just like with individuals and families. Especially when working with couples, there will always be new pieces of context to uncover. For this reason, we have CRT techniques and interventions that we use specifically with couples in relational work.

Let's briefly talk about scheduling with romantic relationship clients. When working with a relationship, at least half of the sessions should be as the relationship unit. Ideally, the first session will be together with subsequent individual sessions. In the breakout sessions, therapists can assess for past and current individual and relational trauma and affirm the absence of contraindications.

After the initial joint and individual sessions, the clients and therapist collaborate to decide how often they hope to meet as a system versus individually. For example, they may prefer two sessions together followed by individual sessions, or they can do more consistent sessions together with fewer individual sessions interspersed. CRT balances relational and individual sessions to provide holistic care to the client system. Individual sessions can offer opportunity for the clients to dive deeper into their selves, discern what contributes to their sense of safety and security, and identify possible blocks for compassion when they may not yet feel ready to share these with loved ones. That being said, the relationship remains the therapeutic client even when meeting individually.

Romantic Relationship-Specific Assessment Features

As relational therapists, we want to understand the client system's strengths, challenges, pertinent history, and the like. In addition to the individual and applicable family-based questions, here are some specific romantic relationship concepts to potentially explore:

Gathering Relational Context

As we say in family systems therapy, context is everything, and assessment is the gathering of context. For romantic relationships, assessment will want to know:

○ How the clients met
○ Their first impressions of one another
○ What keeps them in the relationship
○ How they solve problems, individually and/or together
○ What led them to pursue therapy now

These assess the presence of relational compassion in how this information is provided – are they curt, or are there tones of fondness? Do they rabbit trail in their stories, or are they brief with an exhausted or withdrawn affect? Hearing significant events in their inter- and intrapersonal histories informs the therapist of what relational healing and restoration might be needed. This is also when we begin to reflect with clients using perspective-based language and listen for the relationship's capacity to tolerate different perceptions of events and experiences.

Assess for Client Perspective of Relationship

Seeing the client's ability to cue into another's point of view, including their beliefs, values, and emotional context, is an important part of assessment. The therapist will listen for the clients' ability to receive a loved one's perspective:

• Does the client interrupt others, including the therapist, such as jumping to conclusions as to what the other person thinks, feels, or what they are about to say?
• Are they quick to become defensive or to "go offline," checking out from the conversation?
• Do hardships or challenges in the relationship immediately seem insurmountable or overwhelming?
• Are they able to identify strengths in the relationship and/or in one another? Does the client compliment their loved one, or identify strengths/uplifting characteristics of the other person? Are those conditional or transactional?
• Can the client accept the compliments from the other person, or do they minimize or reject them? Saying, "I'm not like that," or, "Where has this been these past five years?" indicates a lack of compassionate receptivity.

- How do the clients talk about one another's views? Is it viewed as illogical ("I can't believe they would think that's okay; it makes no sense that someone would think like that") or open to consideration ("I don't agree, but I can see where they're coming from")?

As discussed earlier, understanding the capacity that a couple has for compassion for self and another is going to be one of the first steps of the assessment procedure. We tune ourselves into this by listening to their language, and exploring their desire and openness to learning a new way of interacting with themselves and their partners.

Those client perspectives of the relationship can help us understand what capacity for compassion is already present and where some of those areas of growth might be as well. With this lens in mind, here are a few relationship-focused questions a CRT therapist could ask in their assessment process:

Mindful and Meta Perceptions of the Relationship

As we talk about the past and present of the client relationship, we also want to do present moment check-ins. These enable us as therapists to see in the moment what's happening for clients and what their internal processing is looking like. We can look into this by asking: *"What is it like to talk about the strengths of your relationship right now? What about the hardships in your relationship?"*

These questions are related to the idea of shared human experience. It is part of life that we all go through challenging things, and everyone feels differently about those challenges. We also process and integrate these experiences differently. Some people internalize, others write them off as irrelevant, some try to distance and avoid, while others find that set core beliefs emerge from these encounters.

Upon asking this question, the therapist will offer a compassionate response aimed at meeting the client wherever they might be. For example, we might get a response along the lines of *"I hate talking about those, it makes me feel so uncomfortable,"* or *"You know, we've been through hard things, but I believe we've learned from them and I want to keep learning."* If it feels hard and discouraging, the therapist will make space for that, and if the client has a more positive outlook on the challenges they've faced, the therapist will meet them in that space too.

Remember, CRT talks about the problem as an external entity from any one person in the system – the problem is in interactions with self, others, and ideas (including the problem itself!) that lack compassion. Aside from present moment check-ins we also want to ascertain, *"How does the romantic relationship talk about challenges?"* Is it all consuming and insurmountable? Is it only a problem because of their partner? Or is it a challenge they're working to navigate or a space of growth that they're trying to get through together? How clients frame and conceptualize their problems can tell us a lot about the compassion they have for themselves or others.

As an extra note, it's important to keep in mind that with all of these questions we're listening for the client's ability to take the appropriate degree of responsibility for relationship problems (versus blaming the other person excessively or taking on excessive blame themselves). It's the classic "it takes two to tango," mentality – feedback loops, as family systems would say. More often than not in relationships, both individuals are playing a role in the situation or challenge, however the ways in which they may or may not be contributing can look different. While interaction cycles require at least two participants, the contributions might not be 50/50. For example, if there is abuse occurring, the recipient may contribute to the cycle through inaction or passivity (a survival mechanism). This is not held equal to the actions of the abuser as contributions to the ongoing problem.

Ongoing Use of Individual Sessions in Therapy Process

According to cybernetics, people act differently depending on who is present, including their partner(s). When working with romantic relationships, we want to see the system members both individually and as a unit to notice these differences in affect, personality, and potentially information shared. These help us understand the perspectives of each individual outside of the relationship. These also help us as therapists learn more about their individual backstories, families of origin and what significant life events might be impacting the clients. This is important information to know because these pieces of life will inevitably impact the individual, but when we are in couples therapy we're focusing so much more on the relationship. Knowing these parts of the clients stories will help give us the context we need to understand additional relational elements.

Goal Setting in Romantic Relationship CRT

The assessment questions we've looked at also inform the goals set for therapy. We know that it is a therapeutic cliché how often relationships come into therapy wanting to work on "communication." However, the challenges usually go beyond "communication" and how they talk with one another. It is tied to meaning-making and felt connection and intimacy between them. While we acknowledge and affirm the client's perception here, we also use compassion-based skills to see what might be under the umbrella of "communication."

Therapists listen for common desired outcomes between the client system members, even where they might phrase them differently. For example:

- Partner A says, "I'd really like them to understand how it hurts me when they make decisions without taking my needs or wants into consideration."
- Partner B says, "I'd really like them to understand that I make decisions with them in mind; I just don't always check in with them first."
- Therapist reframes, "Sounds like a goal for us is to understand and feel understood by one another, which maybe is missing right now. What a challenging thing to feel! Tell me more about what you hear or see from someone that tells you, 'They get it. They understand.'"

This is also an example of a couple that is holding each other responsible for change – they want the other person to understand. The therapist's reframe pulls responsibility back to each person individually, highlighting that both parties contribute to the current missed understanding. The therapist then poses a present-focused question seeking clarification of how they know they feel understood; this is to help the clients recognize when the goal is starting to take place later. Chances are, in romantic work, a common goal will be feelings of connection and trust. We can always lean on this language compassionately. The CRT couple relationship questions tie into our modality comparison for this chapter – Gottman Couples Therapy.

Modality Comparison: Gottman Couples Therapy

John and Julie Gottman have been foundational in creating digestible, step-by-step interventions for couples therapy. They have completed decades of research surrounding what contributes to building a safe, secure, and connected relationship. They believe that every relationship needs friendship and intimacy, trust and commitment, and passion and romance. Gottman couples therapy takes clients step by step through building a "Sound Relationship House," which has end goals of facilitating shared life meaning, a future they're both invested in, and deeply connecting rituals.

Gottman and CRT have some overlapping elements include the role of psychoeducation regarding bids for connection, repair methods, and points of disconnection in a relationship, what the Gottman method would call the Four Horsemen of the Apocalypse: Criticism, defensiveness, contempt, and stonewalling. The Gottman method also poses some very specific assessment questions for couples and how to interpret them. While CRT will have some similarity in terms of utilizing assessment questions geared toward understanding relationship history and couple disposition, how we ask these questions and the intention behind them shifts:

Table 10.1 Gottman vs. CRT Language

Gottman Goal:	CRT Language:
Listening Capacity: Can we listen to one another?	How much compassionate receptivity do we have for a partner's perspective? For our own perspectives?
Knowing Partners World: Do we know our partner's world?	How does it make sense that your partner had this response? (Compassionate contextualization)
Self-Regulation: Can we self-regulate?	Can we recognize when we need to pause? Can we normalize taking a break for ourselves and our partner?
Accepting Partner Influence: Can we accept our partner's influence?	How can we receive compassion from our partner for our perspective?

In addition to its assessment methods, one of the great things about Gottman's approach is the level of structure the interventions offer. This can be hugely helpful for clients and very beneficial when building foundational communication skills. CRT differs from this scripted response to encourage clients to individualize their responses and utilize language that feels authentic for them. This means leaning into inside jokes, relationship dialectics, and the like.

An example of this would be Gottman's listener/speaker exercise. This is a wonderful introductory communication exercise where couples work on listening to their partner and communicate that by phrasing back to them, *"What I heard you say was . . ."* and then checking for understanding by asking, *"Did I hear you correctly?"* Instead, CRT might ask, *"I know what validation looks like and sounds like to me; what does validation and compassion look like and sound like to you?"*

A Note from Emma: Ironically, the week I sat down to begin writing this chapter, I had a client session where the couple was working on hearing one another and checking that they were understanding each other correctly. They were working on talking about boundaries and validating one another's perspectives. Partner A shared their thoughts and feelings and Partner B responded with, "I felt the same way when your dad crossed that boundary!" I paused and asked Partner A if the response they'd just received felt validating and connecting for the client since from my perspective it felt like Partner B had turned the conversation back on them. My initial assumption was "Oh, I feel like that isn't validating or affirming." However, Partner A responded with "No, that is definitely validating to me! We always validate each other like this. It makes us feel like we're on each other's team." This circles back to our earlier CRT couples question of seeking client perception and using that to inform our perspectives versus us as therapists labeling what that validation or affirmation would look like.

Case Example

Since we spent time exploring couple relationship dynamics and intervention examples in Chapter 5, here we're going to jump right into our case conceptualization to see how these dynamics and interventions would play out in session. As a quick reminder, here are our main intervention categories:

1. Intentional language
2. Compassionate contextualization
3. Disentangling
4. Positive restorations
5. Temporary agreements

Let me introduce our case study for this section of the book. This heterosexual, cisgendered, upper middle class couple came into the office citing "communication challenges and lack of connection." Sabrina, a 37-year-old Japanese-American, has been married to Rob, a white 47-year-old, for 12 years. They have one 8-year-old son. Sabrina and Rob met while at graduate school in New York, both of them getting Masters' degrees in business. Sabrina was on a student visa while she was in school. She and Rob started dating at the beginning of their graduate program and got married after the program finished. They both got jobs working in different technology companies and Sabrina worked her way up into a management position. A few months ago Rob unexpectedly lost his job. Since then, he has been looking for another job and taking over some of the household responsibilities. He has been doing some work around the house and certain chores, although Sabrina still feels like she is doing the bulk of daily house management (cooking, laundry, cleaning) on top of working her full-time job.

The couple comes into the session feeling frustrated with the relationship dynamics they're experiencing. Rob feels like "he couldn't control getting laid off" and now Sabrina is resentful toward him for something he "had no say in." Sabrina feels like she is constantly overcompensating and "doing more than she should have to" which contributes to her feeling resentful toward Rob.

Let's apply CRT to a session with this couple. We've worked our way through some intake material, and conceptualized that this couple has willingness to engage in psychoeducation, and some capacity for compassion for self *(Assess for Client Self-Perception and Introspection)* and other *(Assess for Client Perspective of Relationship)*. We know that both Rob and Sabrina feel resentful toward one another. This is an excerpt from their fourth session; as with previous chapters, the interventions are italicized where used.

Therapist:	So, as we explored a bit in our last session, there seems to be some mutual resentment that you both are noticing in the relationship. Tell me a little bit more about that.
Rob:	I think I feel like it started after I got laid off. It was a really challenging time for us
T:	Rob it seems that feeling some resentment from Sabrina contributes to you feeling disconnected from her. It appears that not feeling that compassion and warmth increases insecurity for you. Does that feel accurate?
R:	Yeah, that does.
T:	Okay, thank you for that Rob. Sabrina, I'm curious, let's talk about this, does Rob's desire for some connection and compassion in this situation make sense?
Sabrina:	Yes, I mean of course it makes sense that you'd want to feel that and get compassion. I want you to feel that way. I just feel like I'm already doing so much, and in fact I'm doing more than I should have too. Like, why should I have to work and also take care of the house? *(hypothetical why question)*
T:	Ooh, let's pause here, because that's a significant question! *(answering hypothetical why)* I hear that Sabrina, and it feels so important to recognize the work that you're doing here. You both are navigating a lot.

S: Yeah, I really feel like there's a lot to try to figure out here. I definitely get discouraged sometimes. I get that he also feels discouraged. That makes sense to me.

T: I bet! It can feel so discouraging and I imagine disheartening to feel like we're doing more than our fair share. Rob, Rob, after hearing that, how does it make sense to you that Sabrina feels this way? (*circular compassionate contextualization question*)

R: It is nice to know that she wants me to feel supported. Sometimes I feel like it's hard for her to care.

T: I hear that Rob. I can imagine that it feels disconnecting.

R: It really does. I promise I'm trying, I just feel like I'm not doing it right. I'm glad that she can see where I'm coming from though. It makes me feel less alone.

T: It seems as well Sabrina, that you feel as though you are trying hard to support Rob, *and* trying to show up for him, while *also* not compromising yourself. (*"and" language*)

S: Yeah, I really am. It's hard for me to balance because I already feel like I'm compensating in more ways than are comfortable for me.

T: Wow, thanks for that Sabrina. It sounds like that's been a challenge you've been navigating. Rob, what's it like for you to hear Sabrina share that?

R: I do know that she's trying to not take it out on me. This isn't what either of us expected, and I know that she's doing a lot. I'd be frustrated if I was in her shoes. (*perpetual opportunity for compassion*)

T: Wow! Sabrina, What's it like to hear Chris acknowledge and see your perspective, even say he understands your frustration? What's it like to know that he recognizes all the work you've been doing and the heart behind it?

S: I'm glad he can see that. I'm glad too that he can recognize the ways in which I've felt frustrated. I know it must feel challenging for him when I seem resentful all the time.

In this section, we see that both individuals were able to see where their partner was coming from and accept that they were feeling the way that they were. One of the pieces we want to be mindful of as well is which partner we lean into compassionate contextualization with first? For example, we see in modalities such as EFT that Sue Johnson would engage with the pursuer first to help them feel ok to pause their chase while she then turns to engage the withdrawer.

In CRT we want to start with whoever "brought the issue" to the table. We want to lean into whoever offered the initial introspection and emotional vulnerability. When this happens, clients are demonstrating receptivity to that emotionality and vulnerability which is one of the most valuable parts of CRT.

When we see this happening in session we want to honor this and let the clients know that when they lean into this part of themselves, space will be made for it, versus being dismissed or invalidated. If we consistently see that one person shares first, we may find that we will reflect on the previous session's work to make sure we bring in the second person more and encourage their thought-sharing process.

Chapter 11

CRT with Ethical/Consensual Nonmonogamy

Working with ethically/consensually nonmonogamous (ENM/CNM) romantic relationships is an extension of work with romantic dyads, not something new altogether. The goal remains to increase compassion within self and with others. Contraindications to treatment remain the same: current abuse, addiction, or affairs.

We are intentionally addressing ENM as separate from infidelity because it is something different entirely. ENM it is the informed and mutually consensual inclusion of more than one party in a romantic, sexual, and/or intimate relationship. Polyamory is a type of ENM, along with polyfidelity, throuple/quads, hierarchically open, closed V, open or closed swinging, and other structures of open marriage/relationship. To what extent the relationship is sexually, physically, or emotionally intimate varies, using nicknames such as parallel, garden or birthday parties, or kitchen tables. The consistent criteria is all parties consenting and the absence of secrecy.

CRT is applicable to both couples shifting to ENM and multiples that have been open for the whole duration of the romantic or sexual relationship. Depending on the structure, as with families, it can be appropriate to work with specific dyads and triads within the system. CRT approaches ENM as a sexual identity or lifestyle, not a kink preference or sex addiction. While some view it as a sexual orientation ("It's who I am, not a choice"), the underlying theme is relational multiplicity as one's authentic romantic fulfillment.

Contextualizing Why People are Drawn to ENM

ENM appeals to those who enjoy expanding their love, sex, family, trust, and commitment. It is not a lack of "completeness" in oneself; research shows that a substantial percentage of ENM practitioners have secure attachment styles. ENM helps people:

DOI: 10.4324/9781003518730-14

- improve relational need fulfillment, particularly not being reliant on an individual to meet one's needs and increasing community connections;
- pursue diversity of sexual experiences/interests and nonsexual activities; and
- foster personal growth, autonomy, and self-insight, particularly coming out of a repressive social system.

These can be part of monogamous relationships, too, with a reasonable amount of emotional nonexclusivity, such as close friendships and personal hobbies.

Formerly monogamous relationships may shift to ENM to fulfill any of the above reasons. Additional logistical reasons can be a partner coming out as asexual or chronic illness resulting in sexual dysfunction. There are other, potentially less healthy, reasons people attempt to introduce it. "Why ENM?" will be an essential early question in the assessment process.

Common Challenges Shifting to ENM

For couples shifting into ENM, let it be a transition! By the time one person brings it up, they may have been thinking and preparing for a while and have already started shifting perspective. Give the partner space to receive the idea. Expecting them to jump on board immediately, fully understanding the implications, may not be realistic. When couples shift to ENM, there are common challenges they may come across:

1. Wanting to change the structure of the relationship without addressing the innate shift in relationship roles.
2. A lack of skills, such as poor communication or poor emotion self-regulation.
3. Low personal autonomy, demonstrating dependence or codependence (see Chapter 12).
4. Differing views of ENM as a sexual lifestyle (choice) versus orientation (not a choice).
5. Potential awakening of other aspects of one's sexuality, including deconstructing assumptions and social oppressions as part of the transition.
6. Attachment crisis – our relationship connection isn't as secure as we thought.

These are not relational death sentences. If any of these are present, we will need to disentangle the assumptions blocking compassion around the issue. ENM may be a dealbreaker to some people, and that is valid and necessary to address, too.

> **A Note from Bethany:** When I have clients express interest in ENM, I always reiterate that trust and communication have to raise a level of intentionality, even compared to monogamous relationships, because open relationships can invite opportunities for insecurity.

In addition to these direct relationship challenges, we must acknowledge the challenges of monogamy normativity, or the cultural assumption in romantic relationships that they will be closed dyads unless otherwise specified. People can experience judgment from communities, professions, family, peers, and even themselves for the choice to deviate from this norm, relationally or sexually. This is an unfortunate byproduct of a sex-avoidant or aversive society with an outspoken history of conservative, monotheistic mores. This is chronosystemic context! We will talk more about relieving oneself and one's relationship of such judgments later.

ENM-Specific Assessment Questions

Regardless of when in the process of therapy the client brings up ENM in their relationship, there are specific assessment questions to address for the topic:

"What purpose does ENM play in your relationship?"

In the words of Jessica Fern, author of *Polysecure*, "When the waters of [ENM] begin to pick up and the emotional rapids of opening up your relationship begin, having your why to remember and return to can serve as the needed life jacket that keeps you and your relationship afloat" (2020, p. 105). It is not essential for all partners to have the same "why," but this may inform the ENM relational structure choice. If any parties' answer revolves around appeasing the other person or curing personal loneliness, this may ring some warning alarms and indicate that ENM is not consistent with their authentic sexual self.

"How does ENM fit with your authentic sexual self?"

Do the clients know their authentic sexual selves? Do they feel safe to identify or explore their authentic sexual self with their partner(s)? Can they identify how ENM is an expression of their authentic sexual self?

If shifting from monogamy, "What changed to introduce ENM as an option now?"

What happened for now to be the time to identify and/or address this? Has it been brought up before, and if so, to what reception?

What about ENM appeals to them? How does this feel like a good fit for their relationship?

Does this impact who is considered the client system?
Is there a specific dyad we will work with to focus on building compassionate security, or more? Working with ENM, all partners can be invited to be part of therapy if it feels helpful for the clients, especially closed systems. Metamours – people who share a partner but are not romantically or sexually involved with one another – are still a mesosystem influencing one another. If multiples are part of the romantic relationship therapy process, be prepared as a clinician to dedicate more time to collect personal and relational histories.

Do they know their ENM structure? If so, what does it look like and mean to them?
What does it mean to them to identify as or practice their particular flavor of ENM versus "curious/open," or a different descriptor? If they do not know their preferred ENM intimate partner structure, how would they like to include that education and exploration in therapy? As a side note, Fern's *Polysecure* also provides an excellent description of several of these and is frequently a recommended co-occurring bibliotherapy text in this therapy dynamic.

What current agreements are in place?
This question also asks about role clarity among the system members. How do they see themselves, their partner(s), and each other's partner(s) in relationship with one another? Is there one dyad that is prioritized? What does that prioritization behaviorally look like? What does secure attachment look like for the dyad/triad/group, such as how is trust is experienced and communicated?
We also will potentially revisit general relationship assessment questions (that, though not specified earlier, can have variations in family therapy, too):

- *What are their personal and romantic values, individually and relationally* (i.e. connection, communication, intimacy, transparency, authority, security)?
- *How do they handle jealousy?*
- *How do they currently regulate and communicate thoughts and feelings?*
- *Where do they notice getting 'stuck' in their relationship?*
- *What are their current problem-solving methods?*

These questions do not need to be asked in any particular order, nor are they to be glossed over. Their answers are potentially significant to how each person validates one another and/or the ENM relationship. Additionally, assessment may take longer when more people are involved. Be mindful of time and financial restrictions and urgency of the presenting problem; it may be helpful to lean heavily on out-of-session data collection from the clients to keep treatment momentum. For example, if a quad client system meets weekly, it would take a whole month of individual sessions between intake and the next group session. It may be beneficial to split sessions for briefer individual sessions, if this is part of treatment for safety checks, as with couples. Lastly, we recommend *Polyamory: A Clinical Toolkit for Therapists (and Their Clients)* by Martha Kauppi, which includes detailed questions and considerations working with ENM client systems.

Intervention Applications

Each of CRT's unique interventions is applicable when working to understand and flourish ENM relationships. To do so requires a few additional details to keep in mind, many of which align with working with families:

- In session, the therapist must track the emotional activation of all members, attending to the most intense and needing emotion to create safety in the room without alienating the quieter emotions present, too.
- It is an option to see dyads within the polycule. If you do, it is important to remain multipartial and balanced with seeing the whole romantic group regularly. Information shared in dyads is considered appropriate to include with other partner(s) not present.
- Track the perpetual overlapping triangles of the romantic relationships. In relational triangles, people are theorized to take on specific roles:
  - *Generators* are willing to identify dysfunction or are most vocal to their distress; as a result, they are often the identified patient or symptom-bearer.
  - *Amplifiers* are reactive to the generator, often turning to the dampener for personal support regarding the generator's stress.
  - *Dampeners* act to reduce symptoms, often perpetuating dependent triangulation and negative feedback loops; reducing symptoms may not solve problems, just cover them.

    Both Amplifiers and Dampeners often want healing to occur as soon and as quickly as possible, which can look like a behavioral emphasis in therapy.

Depending on the relational structure, these roles may be assigned to varying degrees. The role someone takes is part of their context: "*Looking at your history and the roles you've held in family, friendships, professional settings, and romantic relationships, how does it make sense that you take on this particular role now?"* This is compassionate contextualization in ENM dynamics.

Intentional Language

Language clarification, seemingly so tedious, can make a substantial difference in trust within ENM relationships and serve to practice safe overt communication:

1. *Defining Infidelity:* Infidelity is typically linked to secrecy and breach of established rules among a polycule. However, some ENM individuals may have their own definition; we do not want to assume what those are.
2. *Defining Spouse and Marriage:* The meaning of marriage, both legally and relationally often signifying a primary, that may differ among partners. We also must acknowledge that polygamy is technically illegal in many places, including the United States. This can challenge the emotions around perceived illegitimacy among the ENM system when a polygamous relationship wants to be entirely equal across all partners but legally can't, potentially resulting in the loss of life partner legal benefits.
3. *Demand vs. Request:* Imagine a partner telling another, "If you love me you'd let me do this." This is a false dilemma logical fallacy, along with an appeal to pity. Demands can include ultimatums and punishing statements, often made in attempt to control a situation. This can also look like "veto power" over a partner's relationship decisions. On the other hand, requests require vulnerability and care for one's partner's/partners' perspectives. When making a request, use scaling to indicate degree of importance without hyperbole. Be clear identifying requests as well as the demands and contingencies, allowing questions. This will tie with temporary solutions. Ultimately, we would emphasize no one needs to do something in deep contrast to your authentic sexual self. The goal is for one's attitude, behavior and values to be congruent, including in sexual expression.
4. *Ranking vs. Competing:* How do individuals divide their time and energy among partners? For example, if a partner reaches out to you while you're on a date with someone else, what is the response, if any? Does that feel intrusive? How is this conveyed to the other person on the date that allows all parties to feel respected?
5. *Secrecy vs. Privacy:* Privacy is the choice to keep information to yourself that is not harming to the relationship to do so and may be shared

if requested (not demanded). Secrecy is the intentional withholding of information from someone, often for the purpose of power or placating. Secrecy is generally an act of infidelity. How do the partners tell the difference between these for them, specifically? What information do they consider "need to know?"

Disentangling Linear Assumptions and Meaning-Making

There are numerous gaps for assumptions in romantic relationships, including ones specific to ENM. Ask if there are assumptions present about:

- Perceptions of ENM, addressing past breaches of trust, both in the current relationship and previous relationships
- What it says about a person who is interested in ENM. This could include addressing narratives of "not being enough"
- How it could impact (or damage) a dyad to introduce new sexual or romantic members
- Behaviors linked to gender, such as, "That's just how men/women are"
- A person's interests or intentions to act on curiosities, such as that someone must want to fulfill a fantasy
- Rules one person believes would be obvious but may not be to the other
- Redefining trust, including assumptions about how to end a relationship, re-close a relationship, or respond to a request to end a relationship with a different partner
- Sexuality and attachment style, like assuming someone is insecure based on their sexual interests
- Meaning-making of women often having more partner opportunities than men
- Meaning-making of jealousy. We can approach this as a secondary emotion with underlying fears of threat, rejection, abandonment, inadequacy, or loneliness

Positive Restorations

The ideas in this section originated in Jessica Fern's *Polysecre*, a book I recommend to any romantic relationship interested in considering or practicing ENM (and honestly, monogamous relationships, too). It highlights the importance of communicating commitment through emotional intimacy, personal insight, and offering secure compassion in practical demonstrations of love. These include:

- Share personal details about yourself (hopes, fears, plans; good news, bad news, and day-to-day beige news). Track significant events in each other's lives, follow up on these as a form of attentiveness.

- Join in mundane life tasks like laundry, job hunting, errands, appointment scheduling, etc.
- Try new things together, both sexually and nonsexually, such as new hobbies, interests, or foods.
- Dedicate time to one another, brief and extended.
- Collaborate on projects.
- Offer physical, logistical, and/or emotional support in life challenges, such as medical, financial, familial, pet, or technological hardships. Offer validation statements and compassionate contextualization. Be careful to notice triangulation at the same time.
- Express gratitude and appreciation toward one another
- Use nonverbal along with verbal communication to convey attentiveness toward them.
- Ask them: *"How do you know when you are a priority to someone?" "How do you uniquely make someone feel valued, validated, and cherished?"* We don't just want to be loved, we want to be respected and liked!

Fern summarizes positive restorations as HEARTS, ongoing interactions that benefit relationships without formal meetings, as might be practiced in temporary agreements.

Table 11.1 HEARTS Acronym

H	*Here*	Be present, focused on one another
E	*Expressed Delight*	Take joy in one another and one another's interests and successes
A	*Attunement*	How do you "get" one another and show you "get" the other, moment to moment and overall?
R	*Rituals/Routines*	How do you connect, moment to moment and overall?
T	*Turning Toward*	How do you receive and offer support with one another?
S	*Secure Attachment with Self*	How do you offer yourself compassion?

Temporary Agreements

As discussed in previous chapters, temporary agreements focuses on allowing curiosity and giving permission to not have the "right answer" for what works for you or your relationships on the first try. This can be particularly relevant in ENM in the exploration of relationship structures. Instead, we can make recurring commitment to explore together securely and compassionately. Different structures may fit better based on the extent of desired emotional and sexual nonexclusivity. These could be considered a form of boundary negotiation. It is normal for romantic relationships to need to revisit current agreements related to topics such as:

1. Rules/expectations (such as the use of birth control, hygiene, or protection from and frequent testing for sexually transmitted diseases)
2. Financial responsibilities across relationships
3. Hard or soft limits and expected communication around these
4. Identifying triangulation among partners, often through gossip-like communication about one partner with another or putting them in the position of Dampener

In these agreements, it is important to be clear about behavioral and emotional needs throughout the "experiment," such as overlapping positive restorations. It is essential in secure relationships that parties feel safe to identify their wants and needs without judgment.

Remember, temporary agreements can include both "living as if" for the determined time or include brief check-ins throughout, such as through scaling questions. For those who prefer a formal meeting structure (such as to avoid "random" uneasy conversations), RADAR is a check-in system designed to be held monthly, or more often as beneficial (particularly early phases of the ENM relationship). It was designed by the creators of a well-known podcast, *Multiamory*. It's structure holds space for both a celebration of what works and opportunity to discuss hardships securely (Table 11.2).

Table 11.2 RADAR Acronym

R	**Review** the past month of significant events, action points completed or attempted, and what action points are continuing into the next month
A	**Agreed** Agenda of topics to cover and their order. Common topics to cover are: Quality time, Sex, Arguments, Health, Money, Professional work, Household, Travel, Family, and Other partners
D	**Discuss** the topics identified. Practice nonaggressive communication skills of compassionate contextualized reflection (How does it make sense?), identification of one's own feelings and needs, and make requests for new temporary agreements and boundaries on that subject
A	Create an **Action Plan** based on those requests that feel compromising and compassionate for all parties (this is the temporary agreement – *What are we going to try different between now and next meeting?*)
R	**Reconnect** with one another by ending on a positive note with statements of appreciation, compliments, physical intimacy (cuddling, massage, sex), or a fun date activity.

Modality Comparison: Emotion-Focused Therapy (EFT)

Pioneered by Sue Johnson, EFT is an attachment-based couple's therapy model that focuses on increasing emotional security between the partners in order to change interaction patterns. Over the course of three therapy stages, the therapist guides the client system through recognizing their current feedback loop and their attachment history's role within it. The individuals learn to turn vulnerably toward each other, seeking comfort in one another's acceptance of primary connection-seeking emotions. Once they are able to do this with relative consistency, they create a new interaction cycle that is more mindful of one another and one's own underlying needs, now with the security to convey these more directly.

The minimal existing literature using this modality with ENM focuses on non-hierarchical polyamory, particularly nesting partners (those who live together). Consistent with CRT, EFT is nonpathologizing, focuses on primary emotions, and prioritizes creating emotional regularity and relational security through understanding, accountability, and trust, phrased in the language of attachment theory for EFT and compassion for CRT. Both therapy models also utilize the therapist as a multipartial triangulated entity, able to bear the brunt of the clients' emotions while the other partners are dysregulated. They do this by demonstrating compassionate validation responses, providing language to soothe or validate self or one another. Both also recognize the unique necessity in ENM relationships to overtly validate the polycule structure, not identifying it as the problem in cultures that may assume so.

CRT is mindful of attachment styles as part of someone's context but does not heavily emphasize building secure attachment as part of treatment. CRT also has less emphasis on coregulation, instead leaning more into balanced compassion for self and others without relying on the others to regulate one's emotions. Additionally, CRT is less about drawing out the interaction cycle blueprint and more about the recognition of others' perspective/emotion amidst validating oneself – "How does everyone's feelings, thoughts, or actions make sense for myself and my partners in this moment?"

Psychobiological Approach to Couples Therapy (PACT) is another relational modality working with ENM relationships. It is founded in the assumption of hierarchical polyamory, utilizing clear relational boundaries to support and prioritize the health and unique role of the primary relationship. PACT then oversees communication to mutually manage additional partner relationships through these boundaries that are agreed upon by both primary partners. This obviously differs from EFT or CRT, though the communication of boundaries related to trust is always important.

Case Example

Let's jump back to our couple case study from our previous chapter, Rob and Sabrina. As we will explore further in another chapter, they have different ideas about what cheating in the relationship looked like, and there was a significant rupture that happened because of that. Some sessions later, they've conceptualized that they do want to open up their relationship and temporarily agree to try it for six weeks. After six weeks they want to re-evaluate and see how they're feeling.

Therapist:	Okay, so first and foremost y'all, beautiful job leaning into the temporary agreement and figuring out how you both want to approach this. If it feels helpful, I want to see if we can have some dialogue and establish some understanding around linear assumptions and meaning-making?
Rob:	Yeah, I'm super down.
Sabrina:	Yeah, I think that could be helpful for us. I want to make sure we approach this in the best way possible.
T:	That makes so much sense. I can see how intentional the two of you want to be about this. I wonder, how do the two of you feel it would impact or damage your relationship to introduce new sexual or romantic members? *(Questioning linear assumption and meaning-making)*
R:	I think that if I feel like she's putting more effort into a relationship with some other guy than she is with me I'd get hurt by that. Because I don't want it to be a thing where we lose our relationship. And I also feel like if she's having a lot of sex with some other guy, but then not touching or interacting with me at all, that would also feel really frustrating.
T:	I hear that Rob. It seems like for you, you still want to feel connected to Sabrina and want to feel like your relationship with her is a priority even while trying out this new dynamic.
R:	Yeah, absolutely. I know that I'll get jealous and frustrated if I feel like this becomes something that creates disconnect versus an additional layer to the relationship of fun that we can talk about. But also, I have no idea

what will happen because we've never tried anything like this really.

S: Yeah, I feel like a lot of this honestly still remains unknown until we try it. I know that for me I'm worried about the comparison piece, like if Rob finds another sexual partner, is he going to think they're better than me or want to be with them more than me.

T: Okay, so if I'm hearing the two of you correctly, it seems like at the root of things the two of you both have a similar fear – that your partner will feel like whoever might be brought into the relationship will take primary place over your marriage romantically and sexually.

R: Yeah, absolutely. And that makes me nervous because all things considered we've worked really hard to make this relationship work for us and our family.

S: And regardless of how this goes, like my hope is that it just adds something to the relationship and gives us a chance to get the best of both worlds while also getting to meet new and fun people. I don't want to lose Rob, I just want to add something extra.

T: The two of you have worked really hard! I think it also speaks volumes to the care the two of you have for each other that you want to go about this with conscientiousness and awareness. Tell me, recognizing that the two of you have a similar fear, what does being prioritized look like for the two of you? (*Questioning linear assumptions and meaning-making*)

R: For me, prioritization feels like it's in all the little things, you know being the first person she tells things too, knowing what's happening in her life as it's happening and now after the fact, knowing that as a family and as a marriage we come first.

S: I honestly feel similarly. Like for me, I want to feel like I'm not being shunted to the side for other people and their plans and agendas. I want to feel like Rob wants to share things with me and wants to be connected to me.

T: I love this for the two of you. Absolutely! Feeling connected feels so important, and it seems like a lot of this sense of prioritization for the two of you comes down to communication, and really open and consistent communication at that.

S: Yeah, I really think it does. Like for me, if I find out that Rob is telling a new partner all about his life and what's happening and I'm having to ask about it or he's not sharing things with me at all, I know that it will reinforce this narrative of "they're better than me." Especially with the situation earlier this year where I felt cheated on, I know that I'm a little more hyper aware of that.

R: Yeah, I get that, I can imagine that especially since that happened, wanting to feel like you come first relationally feels really important. *(Compassionate contextualization)*

S: Yeah, it really does for me. I really appreciate you noticing that and acknowledging that. I definitely want you to feel prioritized in this as well and can see how it would feel hurtful if I wasn't communicating or being open with you. *(Compassionate contextualization)*

Chapter 12

CRT with Codependence

One of the therapy buzz phrases we hear fairly often is "Ugh, I'm so/they're so/why are we so *CODEPENDENT*?!" A quick online search describes codependency as being emotionally reactive, needy, self-sacrificing to the point of self-sabotage, enabling, and lacking self-esteem. However, this is a surface-level conceptualization. It misses the context and compassion for people who deal with codependent tendencies in themselves or their loved ones every day.

Concrete verbiage surrounding relationship and interactional dynamics have become more mainstream. The lines defining healthy interdependence versus codependency in relationship seem more and more blurred. We've sat with clients who have lamented their codependent nature, and when we've explored this, we have found that their version of codependence means that they want to call their partner or loved one when something big and exciting is happening. They want connection and safety and want others to feel safe as well.

In this chapter, we explore how CRT views codependence as unique from enmeshment or coregulation, compassionately contextualizes it individually and relationally, and therapeutically approaches codependency in conversations with clients.

Conceptualizing Codependence

The popular book *Codependence No More* by Melody Beattie describes codependence as making someone else's problems your own. The best-seller states codependence perpetuates a missing sense of fulfillment, belonging, or safety in each individual involved and thus, their relationship. While we think this is a piece of defining codependence, we also feel that this version gives the impression that codependence is one-sided, linear, or non-cyclical. It does not recognize how people get to the point of taking those problems on, or how codependence hopes to help a relationship last. And one thing

DOI: 10.4324/9781003518730-15

we know about codependence and codependence in relationships is that it takes multiple people to complete the cycle.

When we look at other therapy models, we see that a familiar narrative is stuck, too:

1. Psychodynamic therapy explores the role of perpetuated victimhood from childhood into adulthood impacting relational dysfunction.
2. CBT focuses on directly facing the disparity between perception and reality and setting firm boundaries.
3. Bowenian Multigenerational therapy identifies codependence as lack of differentiation.
4. Structural family therapy emphasizes hierarchy between the codependently behaving individual(s), those they over-function for, and the triangulation with people they push out or pull in to reinforce their dynamic.
5. IFS rejects the overt language of codependence but explores the pattern of internal parts of shame, caregiving, and resentment.

Diagnostically, codependence is often labeled through personality disorders, particularly borderline personality disorder (BPD). Particularly in Western cultures, BPD is steeped in stigma and judgment associated with lack of logical thinking and emotional reactivity. As I write this, I am mindful that men are less likely to be given this diagnosis than other genders and more likely to have the same symptoms labeled as narcissistic. Ironically, these personality types notoriously are drawn together in codependent relationships; they are both styles of interacting that are dependent on one another to perpetuate.

Under the umbrella of codependence, there are many ways this can manifest. One specialist proposes four categories of codependence: (1) the people-pleaser, who silences their emotions and needs with the goal of maintaining peace; (2) the people-matcher, who seeks connection to others by agreeing with them instead of forming or reflecting on their own perspectives; (3) the people-caretaker, who finds their sense of purpose in being giving to others and lacks identity outside this role; and (4) the people-manager, who attempts to control situations and people to avoid systemic distress, despite frequently feeling quite stressed themselves. All four these subtypes of codependence highlight the good intentions that can underlie the behaviors: to create harmony, nurturance, and stability. Unfortunately, this attempt to build a positive homeostasis often results in chronic over-functioning and enabling of others' dysfunction. As a result, the codependent person often ends up feeling overwhelmed, disconnected, drained, and burdened.

Codependence versus Enmeshment

In our efforts to clarify codependence and the role of this in relationships, let's spend some time exploring how codependence differs from enmeshment and coregulation. Since this terminology is often interwoven, we felt it was important to clarify how CRT conceptualizes these concepts and why we want to differentiate between them (see Figure 12.1).

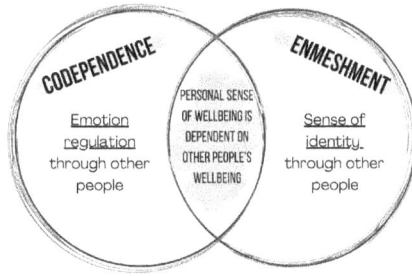

Figure 12.1 Codependence vs Enmeshment Venn Diagram

The biggest difference between codependence and enmeshment is codependence is *emotional regulation* through another person, while enmeshment is *identity regulation* through another person. In enmeshment, identity boundaries between you and the other person become blurred, and our sense of self outside the other person becomes minimal. It's the classic *"I'm nothing without you,"* identity blending we find in enmeshment.

There is, of course, overlap between the two. Both result in someone leaning on another person for their own sense of wellness; there tends to be low distress tolerance or natural capacity to self-soothe. Codependence can be a feature of enmeshment but enmeshment is not necessarily indicative of codependence. They can exist together or separately.

Codependence-Independence Spectrum

Remember the FACES-IV grid in Chapter 7? It uses a spectrum to describe levels of cohesion/connection, ranging from enmeshed to disengaged, and adaptability, ranging from rigid to chaotic. If we put codependence on a similar slide, it would look something like Figure 12.2.

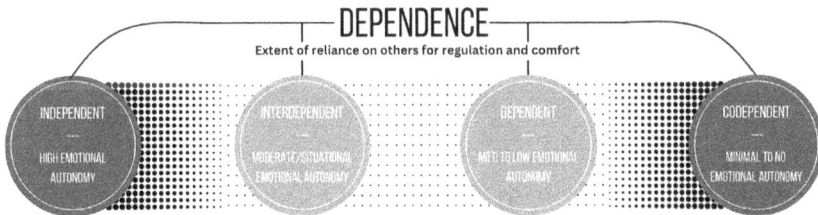

Figure 12.2 Dependence Spectrum

- *Independence* is indicative of high emotional autonomy, or high self-differentiation. While some cultures idealize this, this rugged individualism can actually be detrimental to social functioning as it can also result in low empathy and narcissistic traits of self-over-others.
- *Interdependence* is associated with moderate emotional autonomy. It balances both a sense of personal wellbeing and relational connection to others. Interdependence allows for situational turning to others without the perception of being incapable without them.
- *Dependence* indicates low emotional autonomy. This can be riddled with doubt ("Should I feel this way? Am I overreacting?"), poor self-efficacy ("I don't think I can do this right; I better let someone else do it"), and low self-compassion. Dependence can be situationally appropriate or temporary, but when it is a more permanent structure, it perpetuates dynamics of under- and over-functioning in a relationship. People-pleasing could be considered a form of dependence.
- *Codependence* is minimal to low emotional autonomy. As previously described, this end of the scale lacks faith in oneself to process, or maybe even identify, one's emotions, instead frequently or consistently relying on someone else to lead one through this. Codependence attempts to manage other people in order to manage oneself.

Ideally, all system members get to balance their own independent identity and life while also still feeling like part of the connecting relational unit. The system's cultural context will also contribute to the extent of interdependence and dependence. They will also have the capacity to emotionally regulate themselves and help emotionally regulate others without taking undue responsibility to do so.

Codependence versus Coregulation

Our next relational dynamic we wanted to explore is codependence versus coregulation. The first thing we want to notice is that coregulation is closer to interdependence than enmeshment or codependence. Remember Bethany's soup metaphor? It applies here, too. The idea is that a loved one can provide care without it implying the recipient is incapable of doing the care themselves.

In coregulation, we see the ways in which a partner can be a source of support and grounding. We know that security can be increased in relationships from having an emotional connection to a partner, and coregulation provides an opportunity for that to grow.

To refresh our brains, codependence is a lack of differentiation relationally. We make our partner's emotional experience our own and will often try to manage their emotional experience as well. When we think of coregulation, we may think of a partner seeing distress in their loved one and being willing to lean into it (in theory, this sounds more compassionate in nature . . .). Coregulation is attuning to your partner and through demeanor, tone of voice, and affirmation, grounding alongside them. Coregulation also recognizes that if your partner doesn't ground completely it's not your responsibility to get them to that "calmer place." Coregulation is reciprocative in nature, where all those in the relationship lean into both to take care of one another.

Examples of Codependent Behaviors

Below are a few actions that CRT would consider codependent behaviors. We recognize that context, culture, and meaning-making of the relationship and behaviors can change.

I. Concealing or excusing/justifying the behavior of their focal relationship:

   a. Over-functioning in order to maintain an illusion of systemic functionality

   b. Protecting the other person from consequences of behavior

   c. Distance from and distrust for others who may judge the other person

II. Taking excessive responsibility for the other person's behavior

   a. Fantasizes and obsesses over the other person's problem

   b. Strategizes to attempt control over the other person's problem

   c. Belief that if the other person changed, all systemic problems would disappear

III. Emotional distress

   a. Difficulty addressing one's own emotions, a form of defensiveness tending to shift attention onto the other person

   b. Intense mood swings from high to low (rarely vice versa)

   c. Kept list of resentments and disappointments

   d. Depressive symptoms (increased or decreased appetite and sleep, rumination, decreased executive functioning potentially resulting in lost capacity to manage other parts of life, hopelessness, helplessness, and suicidality)

IV. Tendency to "keep score," related to underlying unhappiness and resentment with the relational imbalance, despite substantially contributing to the imbalance perpetuating

V. Financial problems as a result of these behaviors

Codependence and Shame

Oftentimes those experiencing codependence or stepping out of codependence can feel a lot of shame and embarrassment for past actions and choices. While we want to leave space for everyone's emotional process, we also want to introduce the perspective of using compassion for self and gaining compassion from a partner to promote internal self-healing. Here we reference back to friend-based and parts language: *"This sounds like a part of you that has really valued being a caregiver is feeling unappreciated or embarrassed right now. If your dear friend were having these feelings, how would you respond? What would you tell them? Would you offer a hug or other physical comfort? What do they need to hear right now?"* Instead of shaming ourselves, let's seek to understand and love this caregiving part of ourselves and meet them where they are!

We're not trying to "run away" or excuse away a codependent nature; we're pressing into that part of oneself and journey and recognizing that it *can* be subject to change and growth.

One way in which partners can work alongside us in this journey can be in the role of compassionate accountability. This is one way therapy can be hugely beneficial, for both the codependent individual as well as the partner learning to engage in a relationship with someone who is codependent. Having a space to discuss interactions, work on skill building, while also working on that compassionate partner perspective can contribute to valuable skill building. Furthermore, the therapist takes on the role of accountability manager, so that a partner doesn't have to shoulder more of a responsibility than would be beneficial or healthy for them as well.

Compassionately Contextualizing Codependence

As CRT therapists, we always try to take the compassionate lens. We explore *how* and *why* people act the way that they do and what contributes to those behaviors, emotions, and thoughts. That said, research also demonstrates that there are certain factors that can increase codependent behaviors and tendencies:

1. Trauma
2. Desire for closeness and connection
3. Desire for purpose and sense of fulfillment

A Note from Bethany: I had a client whose mother was easily overwhelmed and would withdraw emotionally and physically. Her daughter learned that if she took on the tasks that overwhelmed her mother – chores and managing her siblings' calendars and emotions – then her mother withdrew less often and for briefer periods of time. In short, instead of learning to cope with her own dysregulation, she learned to cope with her mother's, which pseudo-addressed her own. My client was grown and married by the time I saw her, but she was already perpetuating these same dynamics with her wife. Her wife would also be quick to withdraw when emotionally dysregulated (due to her own trauma history – it's all cyclical!). My client's resulting dysregulation assumed she would feel better if she could just fix her wife's distress. Needless to say, this was both exhausting and unsuccessful long term as her partner received this as a lack of faith in her ability to cope independently. Codependence was staining their relationship but not beyond healing. The relationships involved – with parents, memories, each other, and codependency as a concept – needed to change.

Trauma

Research indicates that abandonment, domestic violence, substance abuse, neglect, and other ACEs can contribute to codependent tendencies in parents, children, and partners. We can also learn codependence by growing up in codependent environments, which can also be a trauma unto itself. As children, our first exposure to what relationships look like come from our primary caregivers. Our understanding of what goes into relationships and what "love" looks like stems from how we see primary caregivers interact. Put simply, trauma is innately relational, particularly family-centric. Therefore, recovering from trauma through intense and intentional seeking of connection can appear as codependence.

Desire for Closeness and Connection

As people, we are hardwired for connection and community, and not experiencing that can feel exceptionally distressing. Beginning in childhood, we try to cope by creating and pursuing all the connections we can in every single way we can. On the other hand, some people avoid closeness and connection based on the assumption that desiring such is the source of distress, not the absence itself. In either case, we see this desire for safety and stability played out in attachment theory. Here we see what different attachment styles look like, and how those can impact our interactions with people and self.

When looking through the lens of attachment theory, it's important for us to recognize the role primal attachment wounds, or traumatic experiences, play in our attachment styles. Attachment wounds from primary caregivers or parents (primal attachment wounds) can stick with us and continue to resurface in relationship after relationship in different ways. One such way is through codependence. It could be said that through codependence, we attempt to soothe our own attachment wounds by trying to fix someone else's. It's the classic, "I try to heal others' wounds as a means to indirectly heal my own." This understandably might seem appealing, though in the long run it can distract us and add more stops on the healing journey.

Attachment theory also connects to fears of abandonment. When we learn that people don't stick around and that people leave, sometimes we compensate by trying to do everything we can to keep them around, even if the ways in which we're doing that aren't as healthy or compassionate as possible.

Desire for connection contextualizes the draw between codependent and narcissistic personalities. Each personality type could be viewed as maladaptive, coping with their past neglect through excessive control. Codependent persons like to be needed and may act as "followers." Narcissistic personalities like to take charge as "leaders." While this pairing is not linear (if one partner is codependent, it does not mean the other is narcissistic and vice versa), it is frequently noticed as it allows a circular interaction of ease: the demanding/controlling personality is not frequently challenged, and when it is, the recipient tend to become more passive over time. However, it could compassionately be reflected that the narcissistic personality is therefore also dependent on their codependent partner to be compliant. They are not as independent and seek more validation and nurturance than a rigid exterior may imply. Therefore, like codependent personalities, there can be healing in compassionate accountability instead.

It's important to remember what registers as codependence or enmesh-ment can change depending on culture, family history, and generational boundaries. What some may view as codependent or enmeshed can be exceptionally typical family interaction from another perspective. It's very important to hold these contextual pieces when exploring these concepts.

Desire for Purpose and Sense of Fulfillment

Along with desire for closeness and connection, people also desire purpose and fulfillment. Sometimes, people can experience codependence from a lack of confidence in what they have to offer. They look for reinforcement and reassurance from others. They often have a lack of self-worth and a lack of space for their own humanness to make a mistakes. This can result in leaning on others to define what is "right" or "correct."

One way in which this can manifest itself is finding purpose through the act of caregiving. Being a caregiver can easily become a huge part of one's emotional world and sense of self – that is to say, one's felt purpose and source of fulfillment. And of course it does! It feels good to feel needed, and humans innately crave meaning and significance! Being needed can also become overwhelming when it feels more obliga-tory than preferential. When caregiving leans into enmeshment, poor boundaries, and an inability to take care of ourselves as we consistently prioritize others, we can run into a bit of difficulty. This can be a learned response or the way someone has learned to interact with the system to "make things work."

We can see a version of this is seen within the addictive system and cycle. This cycle explores how one's belief system can contribute to impaired thinking, which perpetuates coaddictive/codependent behavior. These themes – trauma, desire for connection, and desire for purpose/ fulfillment – are examples of problematic belief systems about boundaries, autonomy, and relationship roles. We say this to help connect the dots for how people wind up leaning into codependence and to help us approach this with a compassionate lens.

When the beliefs, thinking, and behaviors become unmanageable, it circles back to the belief system, either for worse ("I'm just not doing enough!") or, potentially, for the more compassionate better ("Maybe my expectations for myself are unrealistic"). Dismantling these belief systems through disentangling meaning-making and linear assumptions allows the possibility for a new belief and, as a result, new thought and behavior pat-tern that is more authentic to ourselves and our needs.

Intervention Applications

When working with codependence, three CRT interventions will come up most frequently: disentangling linear assumptions of meaning-making, applying compassionate contextualization, and temporary agreements.

Disentangling linear assumptions can be tied to compassionate contextualization as we notice and unknot the past events that lead to the assumptions that codependency makes, such as being unlovable or "too much," enabling behaviors being required rather than options, and the like. Compassionate contextualization can be especially helpful when working with shame responses, as compassion can be a beautiful antidote to shame we feel. In this context, compassionate contextualization could look like spending time exploring:

1. *How did I learn codependence?*
2. *When did being codependent "work" for me in life and relationships?*
3. *What else could be true in those moments when you feel like you have to do the behavior pattern you've been doing?*

Remember, the theme within these is, "How does it make sense that this person behaved codependently in that moment?"

From CRT's perspective, interventions like compassionate contextualization can help bring awareness and gentleness to working with codependence. When thinking about changing codependent perception and behavior, we first and foremost want to decrease self-judgment. It can be exceptionally hard to move forward in compassion when we are perpetually shaming ourselves. Compassion calls us to lean in with understanding, awareness, and acceptance.

To reiterate, compassion does not mean a lack of accountability or repercussions. Instead, it is a way of saying, "Here is what happened, here is why it happened based on the tools I had at the time, and here's how things have been impacted because of it." This is part one. We want to acknowledge the unintentional outcomes. As said by famed addiction author Patrick Carnes, loving bonds can become a prison. While codependence may have had its reasons for being there at one time in life or one relationship, we are also allowed to recognize that it is no longer serving us and may in fact be harming us. We want to self-soothe the distress that comes with these (which may necessitate learning self-soothing at all if comfort was lacking in earlier relationships, particularly parental).

Next comes part two: "Outcomes are not all my fault, *and* (not but!) I did contribute my part. I can also change my part." Here is the shift to temporary solutions: Acknowledge what relationship you want instead (with the other person[s] and oneself), and use temporary agreements to get there: *"What need has the codependence been attempting to meet?"*

In understanding what needs and pains codependence serves, we can shift to better meet those without endangering our lives and relationships. Recognizing and naming what we're looking for and hoping for instead of using codependent behaviors to try to maintain connection can be a beautiful first step in creating new relationship cycles. Furthermore, using temporary agreements to help cultivate new patterns of interaction help us build new habits while approaching change from a sustainable pace.

Modality Comparison: Dialectical Behavioral Therapy (DBT)

Dialectical Behavioral Therapy (DBT) has tons of resources and coping mechanisms which can be extremely helpful when we're working at expressing and regulating strong and intense emotions. One of DBT's areas of specialty is stabilizing and controlling self-destructive behaviors, which we can see surface frequently in codependent individuals and relationships. In fact, one commonality between CRT and DBT would be that both of these modalities embrace and acknowledge that humans have strong emotions that sometimes we struggle to manage. DBT is also similar to CRT in the extent that sometimes we can be embracing two ideas or realities that seem opposite, and yet are true for us. For example, "I tend to be codependent, *and* I am worthy of love and healthy relationships." How CRT differs from DBT is in the mental awareness and abstract thought that can be so valuable when exploring compassion for self and others as a skill. DBT tends to be a great modality for those navigating BPD, suicidal thoughts or attempts, or substance use disorders. For those in the midst of intense mental health growth, the practical skill building and emotional management of DBT would make it possible to engage in the deeper thought abstract work CRT leans into.

Case Example

Rob and Sabrina will demonstrate how CRT has conversations about codependence and codependent behaviors while also working on what *friend-like language* can look like. We've continued on in sessions and learned that Sabrina exhibits some codependent behaviors. They seem to have emerged more extensively after she and Rob moved in together and Sabrina fully committed to staying in the US after her visa expired.

T: So, Rob, I want to hear from you what your perspective is around some of the interactions between you and Sabrina.

R: I just feel like things weren't always like this, but as the relationship has continued, it's been hard for me to know what to do. I feel suffocated at times, like I can't have any space to myself.

S: I promise I'm not trying to be like that, I don't want to be annoying and irritating to him, it just sometimes feels like I can't help it.

T: I hear what both of you are saying, and this feels important to have some conversation around. Sabrina, I know we've talked a bit about codependence and what this can look like. This can be common in relationships especially when you feel like you have to fulfill a particular role. I want to understand, when you reflect on this idea of codependency, *when has being codependent worked for you throughout life? (compassionate contextualization)*

S: I mean I feel like I have to demonstrate to Rob that I'm worth staying with especially because by getting married to him it made it easier for me to stay in the US after graduate school. If I'm not distant from him I can prove that I offer something and prove that I'm useful to him. I feel like when my dad tried to leave when I was younger and was thinking that he would walk out on my mom and I, me pleading and begging with him, and really attaching myself to him seemed to keep him from leaving. So I guess I must have learned then that by attaching myself in every way and leaving as little space for distance as possible that it makes people want to stay.

T: That feels really powerful to recognize Sabrina, thank you for that. That makes so much sense to me! It seems like that early experience with your father informed in your brain that the less emotional distance between you and someone else the better. And even more so, that connecting yourself to them in every single way possible means that they won't want to leave. Did I hear that correctly?

S: Yeah, that definitely resonates with me.

T: What a great example of meaning-making that happens there. That closeness brings safety. That makes so much sense. I wonder if we can explore that a little differently. I want to introduce the idea of *friend-like language*, and have some conversation on how we could use it here, okay? We've talked about what codependence can look like and how we might be exhibiting some of its traits. We also know that Sabrina it's felt really easy to shame ourselves for having some of these behaviors. We want to try to approach this part of ourselves with some compassion, and recognize that it exists for a reason and learned at one point in life that it needed to be present. So when we see or feel ourselves leaning into these behaviors, I want you to work on showing up for yourself as the best friend possible in that moment and give yourself all of the love and affirmation instead of shame for having this pattern. What are our thoughts on that?

S: I like that idea. It almost feels like when I shame myself, it makes it harder to not want to do those codependent behaviors because then just emotionally in general I feel worse. Can I talk to myself however I want in terms of being nice to myself? Are there certain things I have to say?

T: Great question! This can look however you want it too. Sometimes people use terms of endearment with themselves, some people have repetitive phrases that they like to use, and some people like to verbalize the words aloud. The main thing we want to focus on is talking to yourself the way you'd reassure and ground someone you love. For example you could say something like, *"Okay Sabrina, I see you, I see what's happening here in this moment, I'm right here with you let's breathe through this together,"* or, *"There's a reason why I want to act on this behavior right now, it's here for a reason and that's okay. There's nothing wrong with me. It's human to want to be seen and cared for."*

S: I feel like I could also use that language to help me ask for what I need if it's maybe some reassurance or a hug or something.

T: Absolutely, I love that idea and definitely want to make sure we explore that some more. Rob, I want to turn it over to you. What are your thoughts on what we're talking about here. What's coming up for you?

Chapter 13

CRT with Infidelity and Nonconsensual Nonmonogamy

A question we hear and see a lot in media and relationships today is, "Can a relationship recover from unfaithfulness?" People want there to be an easy answer, something that we can know with certainty, a solution, something concrete. For better or for worse, when it comes to infidelity, we don't think there is a one size fits all answer.

Research dictates that there are tons of reasons people cheat/have affairs or engage in infidelity/nonconsensual nonmonogamy. We hear that it was a "one time mistake," or, "it just happened." Sometimes we hear, "they were there when you weren't": Long nights, conflicting routines, struggles in primary relationships, a life-altering event such as sudden loss or change. In the affair/infidelity recovery work we've done with clients, almost all of them say, "The affair was the main event that led to us being here, but the disconnect started a long time before that happened." Infidelity can feel akin to an existential crisis. You question everything you thought you knew, your relationship, and who you are. Compassionately, we can't overstate the pain that can come from infidelity. At the same time, we recognize that humans make choices . . . and mistakes. We do things we regret, and we figure out how to go from there.

In this chapter, we're going to focus on how CRT therapists work with infidelity, and how we view individuals and romantic relationships navigating this relational, and potentially personal, stressor.

Infidelity: "I Know It When I See It"

Infidelity can be physical, emotional, or para-intimate, including singular, temporary, or recurring incidents. While infidelity can be purely emotional or physical, we often see the two go hand in hand.

- *Physical infidelity* can be any physical interaction between person and non-relationship partner in the form of kissing, touching, penetrative

DOI: 10.4324/9781003518730-16

activity, and so on. While this can often be with sexual or sensual intent, that is not necessarily present.

- *Emotional infidelity* can cover excessive emotional investment, often at the exclusion of a partner; secretive conversations or occasions of connection; prioritization of non-relationship partner and their needs over those of the relationship; and the like.
- *Para-intimate infidelity* reference inanimate connections that can feel exceptionally violating and rupturing in a relationship such as addictive substances or processes including pornography, shopping, gambling, or secretive masturbation. We call these para-intimate because there is an illusion of connection in these relationships, such like para-social relationships.

Throughout the chapter, you'll see us use language of cheating, affairs, infidelity, and nonconsensual nonmonogamy interchangeably in reference to the stepping outside the agreed-upon relationship boundaries. The theme is the felt betrayal and breach of relational rules, which is what therapy will focus on in this situation.

So, Why Do People Cheat?

In CRT, we believe a strong factor in the movement outside a relationship is the lack of compassionate connection in existing relationships, including the relationship you have with yourself. Compassionate connection is open, honest communication and having someone who sees, understands, and meets our needs (both surface level and deep/vulnerable) in the ways they can. When this feels unattainable, people may turn to others to attempt to meet them.

We recognize that some people may disagree with this perspective. Not all people crave connection . . . at least, not as they define it. In this way, we are already introducing a language clarification intervention: *"What does it mean to be connected or to want to be connected? How do you know when you are?"*

What's Compassionate Connection?

Compassionate connection includes three core attributes; when any of these are absent, it creates space for infidelity:

1. *Safety in a relationship.* As is commonly understood in romantic relationship therapy, we need physical and emotional safety to let our guards down to be present for ourselves and one another in the ideal way. If we feel that we can't openly share our thoughts and feelings, both joyful and painful, it breeds disconnect and distance. This could be overt

rejection ("Get over it"), or felt inability to bring problems up based on previous responses (negative feedback loops). However, the perception that we cannot have these conversations is a linear assumption. It just means what we've tried so far hasn't worked, not that nothing works.

2. *Relational prioritization.* People communicate priorities in life in how they dedicate their time, energy, and material resources, including finances. Infidelity is not always with a person; it can also be with items apparently being placed at a higher priority, such as professional responsibilities, independent hobbies, friends, or children. When the romantic relationship falls further and further down the priorities list, that can feel like a betrayal, too.

3. *Comfort versus complacency.* Hopefully, a partner is a source of invaluable comfort; a personified place of security and peace. Complacency, marked by apathy and indifference, leads to detachment and guardedness.

We intentionally state the relationship, not a person, may lack one or more of these attributes. This is consistent with our systemic therapeutic lens.

Shame on Me, on You, on Who?

Let's restate the core CRT message: Accountability does not require shame; in fact, we know healing occurs where compassion is present and shame is absent. Therefore, let's start by acknowledging where shame can linger in any role of the infidelity triangle:

Table 13.1 Roles in Infidelity

Role	Possible Experiences of Shame
The Boundary Breaker	Shame for having gone outside the partnership (especially if there is guilt of personal values misaligning with actions); for the secrecy; for damage/hurt done to other relationships, including but not limited to their partner(s); for having ongoing attraction to other humans, particularly if there is fear of ongoing risk to repeating; for missing the affair partner/relationship.
The Boundary Keeper	Shame for staying with the betraying partner or for leaving them; for the longevity of intrusive thoughts ("I should be over it by now"); personalizing and self-blame for affair happening, often perpetuated by others or wider social narratives ("People don't leave happy marriages," "If someone cheats, it's because they weren't getting something at home").

(Continued)

Table 13.1 (Continued)

Role	Possible Experiences of Shame
The "Other" Breaker	Shame for having been with someone already in a relationship ("It's so selfish; they just didn't care," "homewrecker," "other," etc.); for hurting the other partner(s); for not stopping the situation from happening ("You knew they were married; why would you do that?")

We identify this for all roles as a way of reiterating shared human experiences. Additionally, when the participants both have other relationships, people can fill multiple roles at the same time, adding to the complexity! To reference back to a previous chapter, any one of these people can be viewed as the generator, amplifier, and dampener, depending on how they fill and respond to one another or the coming-to-light of the affair. Infidelity can harm all parties involved and be a difficult recovery process from any perspective. In CRT, there is no judgment for ongoing symptoms of post-affair rupture – it is hard for all those involved, and in different ways.

Infidelity Grief

With infidelity, the traditional stages of grief known to psychology – denial, anger, depression, bargaining, and acceptance – are particularly nonlinear. Several will be repeated as the hurt persists even where healing also takes place. An updated version of these stages embraces the complexity among grief: Shock and disbelief; early grief of change; realization of new reality; search for meaning in loss; diminishing pain; acceptance; return of peace/happiness; and for some people, reawakening through a spiritual shift that embraces mortality and suffering as part of life. CRT holds that any kind of grief, including grief for the relationship and life that was or could have been, is nonlinear. That means the healing within grief is on a non-timeline. There is not a set process or duration for the process of grief. Everyone works through affairs and processes pieces of it differently. Depending on the infidelity, the original relationship, additional life factors, and additional contextual pieces at play, restoration and healing varies greatly, even day to day. Working with clients to ask themselves and one another, "What do you need from me today, or in this moment?" is central to communicating those compassionate connection attributes of safety, prioritization, and comfort. The non-timeline reiterates that there is not a designated duration to heal, forgive, or move on in the process of moving forward.

> **A Note from Emma:** I always tell my couples navigating infidelity that the first six months to a year might be the most challenging, and that they could experience a whole host of emotions and feelings during this time. I always preface that having a set expectation of what their grief and emotional journey will look like can be tricky. It adds a layer of expectation that can lead to shame, which is the opposite of what we are aiming for.

A particular aspect of infidelity grief can be remorse. This could include statements such as, "I can't believe I did that; I feel terrible about it." In CRT, we define remorse as the emotional response to acknowledging and owning the pain that was caused. It is the relationship between a person and the pain their actions caused, both in themselves and others. Feeling remorse provides a pathway for compassion for self and partner to take place. When we feel remorse, it provides an opportunity for us to offer ourselves that gentleness as well as demonstrates to our partner that we recognize the impact of our actions. This can help partners feel seen and heard, decrease resentment, and increase their capacity for compassion as well.

Oftentimes, people want to shy away from the idea of remorse. They will question, how can something feel both compassionate and shame, guilt, or regret? However, remorse does not have to be shameful. It is an empathetic recognition of one's harmful impact to someone else. Let's distinguish again, *compassion is the overt presence of accountability without judgement*; it is the opportunity for perspective-taking and growth, even in the midst of hardship and recovery.

Information-Seeking as Healing

After learning about a partner's infidelity, it is natural to want more information/details. The assumption frequently is that we will feel better once we know the what's, when's, and where's instead of the horrors we create in our imagination. Unfortunately, for most people, this is not the case. For some people, it just shifts from visualizing every potential option to holding far too vivid of a mental picture. Knowing more does not make the picture go away; it adds details to the haze. It adds specificity to the rumination, especially in the early stages of learning about the relational injury.

When the craving comes to get details, we recommend personal reflection:

- What is your mind going to do with this information? Is finding answers and getting details about you attempting to control a situation, set more rigid boundaries, or hold yourself responsible for the other person's actions? If so, this can end up perpetuating old patterns of dysfunction and distrust.

- How do you hope your partner feels about sharing this information? Are you hoping for regret, self-flagellation, or something else? Is this coming from a hurting part of you seeking vengeance?
- Are you seeking reassurance of some kind, such as hoping for a reiteration of their vulnerability or honesty? This could potentially be pursued without the details.

It is important to acknowledge to yourself if the details may be more haunting than soothing to know. That can be hard to admit to ourselves because the ambiguity of not knowing is also hard to bear. We can be compassionate about that, too.

On the other hand, it could be said that it is not helpful to know details . . . *yet*. The information can feel helpful and grounding for people who are able to approach the questions with the purpose of gaining context and learning the emotional logic, acknowledging the shared-but-unequal responsibility for both the past and future. With self- and other-compassion is present, this can be a completely different conversation that is far more constructive, rooted in curiosity, seeking understanding rather than repentant confessional.

Rebuilding Trust

If the relationship is in therapy post-infidelity revelation, chances are they are discerning or attempting to rebuild their relationship. But how? Can we really rebuild trust after infidelity?

Long answer short, *yes*.

When there is a relational rupture, often people feel like they don't even know who their partner was in the first place. "How could someone who loves me do something like that?" "How could they hurt me like this?" "Do they even want to be with me?" "How will we ever move past this?" These are a few of the many questions people ask when their trust and perspective of the relationship and its nature are called into question. Throughout the creation of a new connection (because the relationship will never be "like before"), there will need to be intentional efforts to rebuild trust. This will look different from relationship to relationship because there is no one "correct" way to rebuild trust.

Esther Perel, a therapist famous for her work with infidelity, frequently has spoken and published about the core of trust, intimacy, and relational enjoyment when rebuilding after infidelity. CRT embraces her three stages of relationship healing to rebuild trust:

1. *As is so often the case, step one is acknowledgement.*

   This is the ownership of and taking of responsibility for one's choices and behaviors. This acknowledgement fully embraces personal responsibility without justification (i.e. "I know that I made a mistake, but I just didn't know how to get myself out of it once it started," versus, "I made a mistake, and I know that I caused a lot of relational pain"). Acknowledgement starts with the boundary breaker and can continue to include the circular causality contributions from the boundary keeper. Though not necessarily equal, both parties contributed to the dysfunction that included the affair. Being able to own your own part, without taking excessive or minimizing responsibility, can take time.

   With acknowledgement and the ownership of your own actions, you may feel your own shame. It is not the boundary keeper's responsibility in that moment to soothe the shame of the boundary breaker. Here we reiterate the difference between shame and remorse, reflecting on the act of cheating separate from the person: There is more to them than the affair.

2. *The boundary breaking partner takes on the role of the cheerleader and advocate for both the relationship and their partner.*

   Infidelity can be deeply wounding to a partner, and if the relationship wants to move forward, the individual who stepped outside of the relationship has to show their partner that they want to reconnect and be a source of safety. At this stage of rebuilding trust, the boundary keeper may request new, more rigid or "extreme" boundaries or rules in the relationship. These could be an example of temporary agreements, as the new boundaries are not the "forever boundaries." They are for this time of healing. Compare it to healing a broken bone. These new boundaries and rules are the cast on the broken bone, holding it in one place while we heal, eventually returning to greater mobility.

3. *Throughout, practice holding space for continued discomfort or pain.*

   Remember the non-timeline. Often we see that very early on, there is a desire from the partner who acted in infidelity (and sometimes the other partner as well) to "move past it" and not have it "hang over them forever." While we also do not want the pain the linger, we also know it cannot be rushed. And if there is anything that makes an emotion linger, it's trying to make it hurry along and go away. Trying to heal past or through something as significantly rupturing as an affair *takes time*. Rebuilding trust *takes time*. It also takes intentionality. Together, we rebuild the compassionate connection message of "I am a safe and comforting person; you and our relationship are a priority." Trust comes when a partner learns they can continue to feel hurt or discomfort and that the other will be able to make space for their hurt.

Compassion for self and other plays a huge role in this piece of the work, as healing can come just from being compassionate towards yourself and being kind to yourself when the intrusive thoughts or waves of emotions feel more intense some days compared to others. That's ok. That's part of the process.

Engaging in these ideas with a foundation of compassion creates opportunity for people to authentically own their experience and every part of themselves while also learning the skills to rebuild themselves and the relationship in the midst of it. Next, let's see how CRT interventions also address these steps.

Intervention Applications

Aligned with Perel's approach, CRT emphasizes accepting responsibility for one's actions early in the therapeutic process when addressing infidelity. This can start from the very first session as the therapist offers the nonjudgmental compassion statements to the people there: *"Thank you so much for telling me. I imagine there are so many feelings and thoughts around being so forward about this happening."* From here, we learn about the relationship they hope to have moving forward and use the CRT interventions along the way:

Language Clarification and Parts Language

Sometimes infidelity may not be as clear-cut as one partner may believe. What one partner considers cheating, the other may not. In those situations, it is helpful to center back on the undeniable hurt present, whether intentional or not. As a result, healing many include exploring the change in meaning words might have. For example, words like "trust," "loyalty," and "commitment," might have very different meanings post-infidelity. This can be another opportunity for the Venn diagram version of this intervention, marking before and after for each circle and spending time identifying practical applications of these in the overlapping transition time. Clarify the language and the ways in which it might adapt, and use psychoeducation to normalize this process for clients as well.

Parts language can be very helpful when addressing infidelity as it creates space to acknowledge two key ideas:

1. A person acted from a part of them, not their whole personhood ("There is more to them than being a cheater"). Similarly, we are rebuilding trust with that part of them; their other good attributes do not disappear.

2. That part's unmet need is the responsibility of the individual to compassionately heal.

I often refer to parts of us as bits of our past selves that also crave compassion connection within oneself; to feel safe, comforted, and prioritized internally just as much as we hope to experience it in our external relationships.

Disentangling Assumptions

It is so common in infidelity work for people to make assumptions. As I've said before, this is the normal human attempt to fill in the blanks of what we don't know. The struggle with this is, we often fill those blanks in with misinformation. Thinking something does not always make it true. Even when we phrase it as, "It feels like . . .," those are still thoughts or beliefs, which are more helpful to challenge than emotions. On these occasions, we listen for the client's "if/then" statements, and explore other possible reasons or intentions present. We want to make sure we are steering clear of the message that people cheat because the other person "did something wrong." One thing we know for sure is that circular causality shows the other person contributes to the issue, but our actions are ultimately our own.

A Note from Bethany: For context to the audience, I approached writing this chapter as someone who has been cheated on, cheated with, and has cheated in romantic relationships. I can speak personally to how influential compassion is to healing as I have reflected on being in any of those roles. This is not an easy conversation to have with oneself or other people, but it is a conversation people have struggled their way through before. You are not alone in this being difficult or this being done.

Compassionate Contextualization

As previously referenced, compassionate contextualization prioritizes understanding not solely for the purpose of insight but primarily for the purpose of extending kindness to the part of ourselves and partner that acted a certain way that made sense in context. This is true of both the boundary breaker and keeper in these questions or statements:

- *"It is so understandable that it would be so hard to imagine reaching out to them as your source of comfort when right now they are also the source of hurt."*

- *"When your partner first learned about this other relationship, how does it make sense that they reacted the way they did at the time?"*
- *"What past parts of your life come up for you as we talk about this?"*
- *"How did you learn to separate emotions and sex? When or who demonstrated that distinction to you?"*
- *"When you think about this experience that you two are going through, how does it make sense to you that your partner feels shame and hurt?"* *(Circular compassionate contextualization)*

Further along in treatment, we will also compassionately contextualize the benefits each party experienced because of or during the affair. This can function as a perpetual opportunity for compassion ("Now that we see each other and ourselves more fully, we can progress from here"). Here are a few examples of how we can ask this, using language that highlights common human needs like joy or relief:

- To the breaker, *"How does it make sense that you would pursue an opportunity for joy and distraction?"*
- To the keeper, *"How does it make sense that you felt relief when they stopped asking for sex or emotional energy that you didn't have to give?"*

These questions are not asked to give permission or consent to betray. Instead, these questions acknowledge how people are layered beings; we do not want to minimize the complexity of human emotion involved in these relationships:

- *"How does it make sense that they made the mistakes they did when they did?"*
- *"How does it make sense that they feel this remorse now, or came forward with this information when they did?"*
- *"What is it about your partner that, despite the challenges, they are choosing to do the work to rebuild the trust and better this relationship, too?"*

We are not looking for a confession; we are already beginning to practice seeing, understanding, and meeting needs in order to rebuild trust.

Temporary Agreement: Relapse Prevention Plan

Earlier we talked about setting new boundaries and relationship rules as a form of temporary agreements to rebuild trust. These can be placed by either partner as a demonstration of ongoing commitment to improve their compassionate connection. It is true that, more often than not, these rules are placed on the former boundary breaker, but they can apply to the keeper, too. Here are some examples:

o Access to passwords, location services on tech devices and social media
o Disaffiliating with people or places associated with the affair, such as a bar, restaurant, or out-of-work activities. Can also include deleting apps used to participate in the affair.
o Implementation of a curfew
o Requests for additional information about one's routines, such as names of places and people
o Requests for evidence of current whereabouts
o Request STI testing and/or use of sexual protection until test results are clear

As always, agreements will be revisited and more conversations will be had surrounding the couple's needs and wants moving forward. They can temporarily agree to have a plan set for a week, and the next time they're in therapy, they may adjust the plan if desired.

Modality Comparison: Acceptance and Commitment Therapy (ACT)

Acceptance and Commitment Therapy (ACT) puts its core message right into its name: Identify and accept what you can control and commit to make steps to lead a meaningful life amidst the realities of the ups and downs it brings. ACT hypothesizes that with greater psychological flexibility comes increased distress tolerance to work through life's challenges. Increased psychological flexibility stems from a strong sense of oneself including mind, body, and soul, such as self-awareness and congruence between stated values and behaviors.

When looking at CRT and ACT we see that there are some similarities between the two modalities. Both these modalities believe in the acknowledgement of emotions without judgment. They also both have an emphasis on mindfulness, and diffusion as far as "we are more than our thoughts and feelings." Both modalities are also present-focused while also being mindful of context (the influence of the past, present, and future in current decision-making).

There are also some differences we want to make note of. One element of ACT is an acknowledgment and appreciation of pieces of life and emotional experiences. With CRT, we don't require appreciation, just understanding and acceptance with what happened. ACT also believes in embracing emotional pain and hardship as a part of life. CRT believes that while discomfort and pain do happen in life, it is necessary that we differentiate between pain and discomfort in clients. Feeling uncomfortable is different than being in pain, and in CRT we focus on embracing tolerance of discomfort over perpetual emotional pain. We believe that introducing more compassion for self and partner can contribute to less emotional pain and more compassion in the face of discomfort.

Case Example

As you've continued to explore Rob and Sabrina's relational history, you discover that over the course of the relationship the couple has had a challenging time expressing their needs and wants to one another. Since the couple married after graduate school, they have felt that they "didn't have time to explore life outside of school" and "see what the world had to offer." They are committed to one another and wanting to make things work, but feel that their relationship is "stuck in a rut." They have tried to have conversations about leaning into an open relationship. You discover that an area of rupture in the relationship is that Sabrina feels Rob cheated on her in the early stages of conversations around the open relationship by having conversations of a sexual nature with potential partners. Rob feels like they had conversations about this and doesn't view himself as having cheated. He also feels like the agreement they came to "wasn't fair" in the first place because Sabrina had a lot more sexual partner opportunities than he did.

Therapist:	So Rob, tell me a bit more about your perspective on the relationship rupture surrounding conversations with other people?
Rob:	I just get really frustrated, because I don't think I cheated. I don't understand how she can see it that way.
Sabrina:	What do you mean? How is that *not* cheating? You were literally sexting with other women you were trying to get something set up with!
R:	Okay yeah, but nothing happened, so it's not cheating.
T:	It seems like the two of you might have different perspectives on what qualifies as cheating within a relationship. Let's take a minute and explore some of the meaning-making happening here. Sabrina, tell me what comes to mind when you think of cheating? What does that entail?

S: For me, cheating absolutely isn't just physical things.
        I totally believe that cheating can be emotional, or men-
        tal. I know nothing physical happened, but the conver-
        sations that were had very much had emotional and
        sexual connotations to them which takes them outside
        of the realm of normal.

T: Hmm, so for you Sabrina, cheating seems to not just be
        physical, but also emotional or mental and can include
        interactions that happen through technology? *(disentan-
        gling meaning making)*

S: Most definitely. That's why it feels so hurtful, because
        in my mind he absolutely violated the boundaries of the
        relationship.

T: So Rob, we've heard and clarified what cheating means
        for Sabrina. What does that look like and mean for you?

R: For me I just think that because nothing physical hap-
        pened I didn't do anything bad. I just had conversa-
        tions, but didn't do anything in person so I protected
        our relationship.

T: Hmm, so for you Rob, cheating really contains things
        that are physical, and for you it felt like you didn't
        go outside of the relationship since nothing physical
        occurred. Am I hearing that correctly? *(disentangling
        meaning making)*

R: Yeah, that's what I feel like. So I feel like I wasn't disre-
        specting my marriage to Sabrina by doing so.

T: So both of you had very different ideas about what
        cheating was and what that meant. There's frustration
        and hurt that the two of you are experiencing for differ-
        ent reasons here. I wonder, Rob, based on Sabrina's life
        experience, and her conceptualization of what cheating
        means, how does it make sense that she would feel hurt?
        (compassionate contextualization)

R: I mean, I guess I can see why she feels hurt, but I still just
        don't agree with this whole idea and her way of viewing
        things.

T: I hear that Rob. It makes sense to me that based on how
        you view and conceptualize cheating, it is hard to get on
        board with Sabrina's perspective. I also see you trying to
        hold space for a perspective that is different from your
        own. Rob, cue me in, what is contributing to it feeling

	challenging to lean into compassion for Sabrina's perspective? (*relationship reflections – when compassion is missing, steps A, B, and C*)
R:	I don't know, when I think about her perspective, I feel really guilty and like I'm a bad person who screwed up our marriage.
T:	Thank you for sharing that Rob, and for leaning into that introspection and vulnerability. It seems that for you, having compassion for Sabrina's perspectives brings up a lot of hard emotions.
R:	Yeah, I just feel like a failure if I think about it too much.

We see here that Rob's compassion resistance was due in part to his fear. He felt uncomfortable with emotions of shame, guilt, and remorse. Leaning into compassion for Sabrina led to Rob having to confront those feelings about himself and his actions. In this case, understanding the source of compassion resistance, why it might be missing, and disentangling made it possible to better offer compassion to the underlying emotional pieces of this aspect of the couple dynamic.

Part IV

Sex Therapy Application

Chapter 14

Compassionate Relational Sex Therapy

One of the areas of therapy becoming more socially focused on is sex therapy. As authors we are exceptionally passionate about this area of work because, even in the field of therapy, there is still a lot of sexual misrepresentation and misinformation. We wanted to dedicate a section of this book to CRT in the context of sex therapy, sex, intimacy, and trauma, sexual judgment, and kink. There is so much more detail we could go into on almost all of these ideas, but our hope is that this introduction will provide readers with some essential information and the foundational tools for approaching these topics with clients compassionately and with nonjudgmental curiosity.

Compassionate Contexts of Sex and Intimacy

Here is a message that we want to make undeniably clear: Sex and intimacy look different for everyone. What looks, feels, sounds, smells, and tastes like sex, intimacy, and enjoyment to one person is exceptionally different than what it can look like for another person. *This is not only normal, it's _wonderful_.* Unfortunately, we are raised with social messages that sex and intimacy are one and the same, and they look a certain way when done "right." *This is simply untrue.* We are indirectly or directly told how our bodies "should" engage in sexual interactions, often leaving our unique interests untouched. *How disheartening.* Many people share this challenge in themselves and their relationships, often without knowing why. CRT sex therapy emphasizes sexual acceptance, disentangling sexual assumptions, educating about sexual myths, and compassionately reflecting how it makes sense we have the sexual challenges that we do, all while allowing parts of ourselves to become friends (and lovers) with one another.

DOI: 10.4324/9781003518730-18

A Note from Bethany and Emma: We will try *so hard* in this chapter not to tangent or "get preachy" about the societal shortcomings that have led to sex being such a source of erroneous meaning-making, shame, and distress for so many people, particularly in the United States, where both authors are from. Please bear with us as we do our best to balance educating and advocating, both as writers and therapists.

Sexual Acceptance as Compassion

In compassion-based language, sexual acceptance is the application of self-kindness via nonjudgmental curiosity toward one's sexuality, mindfulness of one's body, and the shared human experience of sexuality as a part of one's personhood. Personally and professionally, we have seen shame narratives be so much more present in our sex lives than we consciously realize. Body image is a prime example of this, heavily influenced by social messages that praise youthfulness as an ideal despite its innate temporariness. Similarly, embracing how our bodies function, what our bodies like, and how they work can be a challenge in and of itself.

In CRT, we want to intentionally contradict shame narratives by disentangling assumptions and leaning into the strengths of human bodies. Corrective psychoeducation regarding shame-based or misinformation-maintained myths play a crucial role in creating space for sexual self-acceptance by dispelling untrue or harmful narratives contributing to lack of acceptance or comfort around the topic or practice of sex and sexuality.

Sexual Psychoeducation and Dispelling Myths

More than ever, the spread of misinformation is socially rampant; it is also unnecessarily challenging to discern what is true or not when formal education sources do not provide essential information, including about sex, intimacy, and sexual health. Many clients come with years of misrepresentative narratives, painful messages, false information, and lack of awareness of how their bodies function and exist in sexual spaces. The amount of times we have had women ask, "Is this normal?" is more than we could count.

As CRT therapists, we are responsible for having scientifically accurate and updated information. The confusion, apprehension, self-disgust, and fear based on a lack of scientifically accurate information is too common a starting point in therapy. Especially in the realm of sex therapy, we cannot perpetuate narratives that are harmful and untrue. One way we can begin our sex therapy work with clients is by reiterating the six principles of sexual health (consent, nonexploitation, honesty, shared values, protection, and pleasure). This is frequently the first time they have heard about these, let alone talked about them with each other! Let's appraise an overview of some of the most common ill-informed narratives that may need reconstructing:

1. Biological sex education is sufficient.

False. The majority of sex education provided in the United States is abstinence oriented, meaning it is more heavily focused on avoiding sex than having safe, let alone enjoyable, sex. What education is provided, if any, tends to be biologically focused, or merely a review of the parts of the reproductive system, potentially even of only one sex. Not only is this cis- and hetero-assuming, it also provides a very narrow definition of sex (penetrative) and offers little to no discourse to encourage curiosity. Worse, it may discourage questions or conversations about sex at all. This perpetuates two false narratives: That sex education is more of a lecture than a conversation, and that by not addressing something uncomfortable, it will eventually go away on its own. Ask anyone who has gotten an STI . . . no, it probably won't. Avoiding conversations about sex does not make the topic leave; it just makes the topic feel unsafe. At that point, the person is more likely to turn elsewhere for answers.

2. People can learn what they need to via social media, television, books, etc.

Another falsehood. Over the past generation, the internet has brought an onslaught of social media and television "expertise" and unbridled access to sexual information and material, including pornography, unlike ever before. More people have a platform to present sexual *opinions* as sexual *facts*. These sources often portray a narrow, frequently unrealistic, perception of sex and intimacy. Fantasy smut made a recent resurgence in popularity, and for good reason – it's sexy! However, it can also misrepresent sexual expression, preferences, and consent, or fall into tropes about desire, pleasure, and, frankly, what the human body is capable of. *Fifty Shades of Grey* brought kink to the forefront of sexual conversations while also gravely misrepresenting the community by its lack of consent conversations or sense of safety between characters. It's probably not realistic for me to expect that my very human partner will always have a relentless desire for or magically imprint with me. Chances are low that I'll always give him an instant erection with the slightest touch to his flaccid member or bring her to orgasm by stroking her nonexistent fae wings. All we're saying is that we'd be remiss not to mention how these resources have changed the way we view and talk about sex and fantasy, while still missing essential parts of the conversation.

A significant example of this is the use of pornography for sexual education. A survey completed in 2022 found the average age of initial exposure to internet pornography is 11–12 years old. It can be argued that pornography is a space of individual or mutual exploration and empowerment. However, the audience's maturity, purpose, and frequency of its exposure matters. While it can be used as an eroticism aid, when it is included in a relationship without the consent of all partners, it could be considered infidelity.

In the previous chapter, we talked about three types of infidelity: physical, emotional, and para-intimate, which is engaging in a relationship with a person or practice (such as substance abuse or process addictions) that excludes or rejects our main relationships. We refer to pornography as "para-intimate" because it gives the illusion of a relationship with the observed participants. Porn filmography frequently uses angles and language that enable the watcher to imagine they are part of the action or to give the appearance of the exchange being real rather than a performance. Therefore, while it can be an intimate interaction, due to the nature of the interaction often being purely technological, the connection is one-sided. And like other addictions, its use can become compulsive and a renewed source of shame instead of pleasure.

3. Pleasure is optional or even problematic.

One more not on this list, and not the most ideal message we receive as sexual individuals. Based on puritanical roots, pleasure-based sex has been viewed through a lens of shame. We see this in socialized judgment toward sex work and perpetuating the falsehood that masturbation is evil or dirty, even a form of self-abuse. For women in particular, sexual pleasure is viewed as unsavory, a further dirtying of your already morally questionable genitalia.

Imagine the heartfelt shift that could happen if sex and masturbation was embraced as bodily exploration and a normal part of childhood, adolescence, and adulthood. Because it can be! Masturbation is about learning what you like, and the lack of information women get about their own bodies related to sexual pleasure prominently contributes to orgasm inequity and lower self-advocacy in sexual experiences. This is particularly present where most forms of curiosity are discouraged as deviant. Even the word *pleasure* is uncomfortable for some people, such as those raised in conservative religious environments that rebuke relishing in sexuality as a salacious mix of lust and gluttony.

Pleasure also means so much more than masturbation or orgasms. It covers fantasy, desire, arousal, and mindfulness to the physical and mental stimulation of the present moment. Everyone views pleasure differently, and what is pleasurable to one person might not be pleasurable to another. Don't assume everyone wants more orgasms. In fact, most of the time, we hear people say that they want more connection, touch, and physical engagement, and that more orgasms are lower on the priority list, especially as we age. Pleasure changes over life, just like many other aspects of ourselves. However, it consistently can remain a priority personally and relationally for the sake of life satisfaction.

4. Consent is optional, unimportant, or persuadable.

An emphatic and outright NOPE to this one, while also recognizing where this misconception comes from. Consent is essential in sexual enjoyment. There is also an education gap surrounding how to talk about consent and what authentic and uncoerced consent feels like in our bodies. Depending on the community, context, and sexual interaction there can be different approaches to consent. For instance, clarifying the difference between overt consent and implied consent begins with understanding the relational safety that must pre-exist any kind of assumption of consent. Even then, it remains an assumption. For example, response anxiety (the felt pressure to say yes to a partner's sexual initiation at all times) is a real problem as it builds disconnect and potentially resentment about a partner without even hearing their input! These assumptions can be rooted in cultural pressures, such as "duties" to a spouse (context!), and are actually not espoused by the sexual partner.

By now, we imagine the readers know what we do with assumptions – we check in! The difference between an assumption and an educated guess is checking in. Similarly, consent can be withdrawn at any time, including mid-intercourse, and be valid. All individuals participating in a sexual encounter should want to be there and feel that they can leave at any point they want without repercussions. CRT sex therapy can include conversation of what overt consent looks like in their relationship, approached as a temporary agreement, even using humor to lean into what comes most natural to the individuals in the sexual relationship. We'll go into more detail about consent in the next chapter.

5. Sex is "just sex."

Also false, in so many ways. There are many facets to sex and one's sexuality, both physically and emotionally:

Facets of Physical Sex: Sexual Response Cycle

First, let it simply be said that there is so much more to sex than a penis entering a vagina. Not only are penetration or either of these body parts optional, there are steps both before and after. These are called the sexual response cycle. This includes excitement/arousal, which some would call foreplay or before-care; plateau; orgasm; and resolution, or after-care. When providing psychoeducation about these, it's important to differentiate pre-stimulation desire, bodily arousal, and post-stimulation desire and explore what these look like for each person and in their relationship. Particularly among neurodivergent minds, people can experience challenges at any or all of these stages, often based on assumptions of expectations and linear assumptions. Even the way the cycle is phrased can be heard like steps 1–4. However, CRT compassionately normalizes and encourages a different narrative, such as stage 3 being a part of the process rather than the goal of sex, and that any stage can be returned to after moving to another. Emily Nagoski has written multiple excellent texts on these ideas and their influence in sexual relationships in her texts *Come as You Are* and *Come Together*; we recommend these for both clinicians and clients alike!

One of the biggest predictors of sexual fulfillment and longevity in relationships is whether or not there's cuddling and time together after sex. Sometimes clients have received past messages (directly or indirectly) that desiring foreplay before sexual activity or wanting time to enjoy their partner's presence after sexual intimacy makes them needy or high maintenance. In CRT, we want to disentangle these narratives while also leading clients into compassion for this part of their sexual selves: *"Having needs does not make a person needy, and even if it did, why is it bad to need connection?"*

Facets of Emotional Sex: Circles of Sexuality

The Circles of Sexuality intentionally shifts clinical language to overt sex positivity in conversations about a person's sexual functioning. This included flipping the script to be more focused on positives and strengths of a person than medical terminology rooted in dysfunction or reproductive purposes. Picture a flower-like ring of circles, with one idea at their center (see Figure 14.1).

The flower "petals" that make up one's sexuality are:

o *Sensuality* (awareness of bodies, such as body image, sensory stimuli, our erotic voice, and physical attraction).
o *Intimacy* (physical capacity and emotional need for shared closeness with someone, including oneself).
o *Sexual identity* (sexual orientation, gender identity and expression, and alignment of these with biological sex).
o *Reproduction and sexual health* (factual understanding of different sexes' body parts, internally and externally; their purposes in both pleasure and reproduction; accurate comprehension of physical acts of sexuality, like intercourse; hygiene's impact to sexual wellbeing; correct information about contraceptive options and sexual safety; and sexual health decision-making).

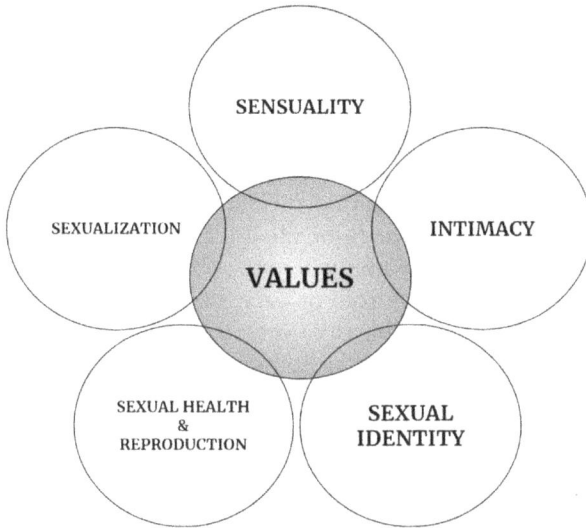

Figure 14.1 Circles of Sexuality

o *Sexualization* (how sex influences your relationship with someone else
  positively [flirting, seduction] or negatively [exploitation, manipulation,
  harassment]).

In the center is a person's sexual values. These values interact with other
aspects of one's identity – spirituality, ethnicity, family, economic perceptions, and geographical region. How a person sexually explores themselves
and other people is informed by the other values. This contributes to someone developing and determining their sexual attitudes and activities.

The sexual response cycle and circles of sexuality are highly relevant
to CRT both as potential psychoeducation tools and to normalize the
immense complexity that sex can pose for people personally and in relationships. It also can provide language for clients in sexual relationships to
talk about specific ideas and perceptions within the topic of sex rather than
become overwhelmed by the topic overall.

6. Sex therapy is about having more, better sex.

We can give half credit to this one. Yes, we want it to be better, but how
that looks is unique to each person and relationship. It will not necessarily be more. Some people have low libido ("sex drive") or identify with
asexuality (minimal sexual attraction) or aromanticism (minimal romantic
intimacy desire). One of the main reasons we see romantic relationships in

therapy is erotic mismatch and feeling like their sexual needs aren't being met. Holding space for both partners to express their underlying feeling, often of disconnect, helps validate perspectives in the relationship by normalizing and offering nonjudgmental acceptance for the varied arousal and desire.

CRT sex therapy is more focused on creating authentic, safe, informed sexual interactions full of nonjudgmental curiosity within oneself and with others. We do this by intentionally increasing mindfulness within the relationships to give compassion where there are challenges, which builds safety. We de-emphasize the role or necessity of penetrative vaginal sex and embrace other forms of pleasure-oriented activity and intimacy building, such as sensual or sexual touch and means of relational connection. Oftentimes, we see clients so desperate to fulfill the cultural, social, or religious role of penetrative sex in a relationship or marriage, that all other pathways to intimacy get overlooked or undermined. As CRT therapists, we hope to encourage and empower clients to discover their own erotic voice – permission to be a sexual being – and help them discover what their pleasure looks like and what their bodies love to do.

Compassionately Communicating Consent

One of the pieces we of course want to highlight is the role of consent and how that plays a role in removing sexual judgment. Consent is not a one-time "yes" (or "I do"), nor does it protect a "yes" said under coercion or felt/perceived pressure or expectation. Instead, it is a continuous and necessary part of communication, interaction, sex, and intimacy. We want to reinforce once more that consent is a foundational pillar of trusting relationships. As therapists, we need to ensure that clients feel emotional, physical, and mental safety in the relationship to freely, willingly, and frequently give or not give consent. This again relates to felt role obligations and response anxiety, such as agreeing to an act for fear or worry about how the other person will receive a situational "no" – that is to say, how they might be judged or rejected for it.

Here are a few specific subsets of consent to potentially discuss with a partner:

1. Consent to have sex-based conversations and stay mentally present throughout.
2. Consent to meet physical sexual needs/limits (such as accommodating autoimmune disorders or limb differences that contribute to comfort, sensation, and movement or autoimmune challenges that contribute to how our bodies show up, what we want to do and can do, and boundaries we want.

3. Consent to communicate known sexual preferences and areas of curiosity.
4. Consent to sexual trial-and-error in the ongoing learning process.
5. Consent to communicate sexual restrictions, hard and soft limits, physical or mental. This includes where we feel comfortable compromising or not compromising.

These do not have to be learned over a single, intense conversation. It can be flirtatious, silly, and another reiteration of compassionate nonjudgment between partners. Communicating these to partners, and having partners receive them, contributes to building a compassionate and trustworthy foundation in sex and intimacy.

Points of Consent-Based Mindfulness

As always, numerous contexts impact giving and communicating about consent. Here are five to consider:

1. *Communication and advocacy fatigue.* Sometimes the work, effort, hurt, and frustration that comes from continuously having to convey, describe, advocate, and confirm understanding about how our bodies work, what they need, what we like and what we can do . . . can be absolutely exhausting. So many people experience great discouragement in this. It can easily lead to insincere consent rooted in response anxiety/apathy. We recommend learning the verbal and behavioral cues of this stage in yourself and partners to learn when to step back and lean on other known intimacy-builders.
2. *Family, cultural, and religious/spiritual influences.* These overlap with sexual disgust and lack of sexual vocabulary or known possibilities. If the first step of consent is building comfort around sexual language and bodily familiarity, then that is where we will compassionately begin, catching any potential judgment about ignorance with compassionate contextualization.
3. *Nonjudgmental conversations will not necessarily lead to participation.* The goal of these conversations is not to convince the other person, but to build a bridge of understanding. Consent is essential for all participants, and if one partner has a fetish or fantasy that their partner is not agreeable to, we can compassionately process that and discuss alternatives.
4. *Erotic versus relationship security wants are different.* If someone enjoys being demeaned sexually, that is the only context they give consent for that relational dynamic, unless they specify otherwise.
5. *Erotic fantasy is not the same as erotic desire.* As part of sexual curiosity, we can discuss what activities someone wants to try participating

in versus those that can remain in cognitive fantasy, where the person remains fully in control of the script of events.

Being mindful of these aspects of consent can help the conversations go better with greater compassionate understanding.

Questions About Consent

When it comes to sex and intimacy, compassionately navigating these conversations can seem precarious. Here are some questions we use when exploring this with clients:

- "If I have a question about ____, how would you prefer me to ask or not ask?"
- "What helps these conversations feel a little more safe to have?"
- "How does it feel best for us to approach this?"
- "What role or emphasis would you want this to have on our communication and interaction?"
- "If I need to check in or clarify about something, how would you like me to do that?"
- "How would you feel about us selecting a 'safe word,' of sorts, that lets me know when we have reached or crossed a limit for you?"

These can be demonstrated by the therapist in session and be used as a temporary agreement for the clients to practice outside of session.

Lastly, it's important to recognize that sometimes, no matter how we approach it or how intentional we try to be, people can still just feel frustrated and discouraged with their sexual situation. Compassion within that is also invaluable. It is an example of perpetual opportunity for compassion as we grant understanding about the ongoing challenges.

Physical and Psychological Contributors to Sexual Distress

All this being said, the belief in and meaning-making of any of these myths contribute to sexual distress. Sexual distress is personal or relational distress via physical, emotional, and/or mental perturbance, and/or value/identity-driven incongruence impacting the ability to authentically and wholly participate in sex. Almost every individual experiences a form of sexual distress, some more than others. Similarly, as is true for other subjects, what is sexually distressing to some people may not be to others. In a relationship, if it is distressing to any partner, it will need to be addressed for how it impacts the relationship.

Table 14.1 Sexuality Stressors

Physical Stressors	Psychological Stressors
o Genito-pelvic pain o Medical trauma o Sexual trauma and/or violence o Hormone changes, such as those from aging or hormone replacement therapy (HRT) o Body changes (temporary or chronic) o Bodily feeling dirty or grimy o Erectile Dysfunction o Vaginismus o Vulvodynia o Premature ejaculation	o Managing personal relationships (families, children, partner[s]/spouse) o Managing professional responsibilities o Feelings and beliefs about sex and intimacy o Lack of physical sensation during sexual or physical engagement o Overwhelmed by life tasks and obligations o Shame due to past sexual choices or behaviors o Socialized discouragement from exploring one's sexuality o Body dysmorphia o Assumptions about sexual roles, such as being a heterosexual male who enjoys anal play

Aspects of life that contribute to sexual distress are called sexual compressors, or detractors. As is often the case, these can be both the source and symptom of life stressors. These are physical and psychological symptoms; some are both (anxiety, exhaustion, etc.). Table 14.1 lists a few common physical and psychological sexual stressors.

Interestingly, some stressors can be both a sexual motivator (factors that contribute, increase, or facilitate arousal, eroticism, and desire) as well as a sexual compressor (factors that decrease, distance, contribute to sex and intimacy feeling more challenging or less appealing for us). For example, when professional demands are stressful, some people seek sexual outlets to release those pent-up feelings; other people avoid sex as another form of demand on their body and mind. Since these factors are different for everyone, we don't want to assume what may or may not be contributing to sexual distress for our clients. Use nonjudgmental curiosity to allow them to inform us of what their sexual distress looks like for them.

Sexual Grief

A distinct form of sexual distress not talked about nearly enough is sexual grief. Sexual grief is the emotional processing of felt loss related to one's sexual self, past, present, or future. This could focus on narratives of ourselves, our bodies, our partners, our sexual engagements. It can also be messages received from larger societies or communities (purity culture), from painful or nonconsensual experiences we encounter, expectations ("I thought it would come naturally"), and disappointment ("I thought it would be different and that I'd feel better after"). Per CRT, the grief is usually rooted in incongruence between our internal sense of one's circles of sexuality versus external experiences or messages.

Relationally, we want to help clients distinguish grief and rejection. Allowing them to confront, acknowledge, and speak to the ways sex and intimacy are not what they expected is vital. Within CRT sex therapy, part of the work that we do will be compassionately disentangling the navigation of anger, woundedness, betrayal, despair, and suffering that grief can bring. Grief wants to tell a story, and showing it compassion is one of the ways in which we can begin to hold it differently. This is one example of how CRT approaches sex therapy differently than other common clinical approaches.

Common Clinical Approaches to Sex Therapy

Before going into a comparable systemic approach to sex therapy, let's first acknowledge that sex therapy models historically have been more physiological and behavioral, such as PLISSIT and Sensate-Focused. These models emphasize growing a tolerance (maybe even a growing comfort) to physical touch and sexual intercourse, which can also be appropriately overlapped with CRT through mindfulness, psychoeducation, and temporary agreements.

PLISSIT

PLISSIT is an acronym of steps when providing sexual health care. The steps are sequential, progressing from one to another, though some clients will only need one, two, or three of the steps and not necessarily all four:

Table 14.2 PLISSIT

Permission	Clinicians must give and receive permission with the client to seek comfortability around this topic including permission to ask questions and voice worries bilaterally – both the client and provider have space to express curiosity and concerns.
Limited Information	Clinicians provide specific information and resources regarding precise questions from the client. This differs from the "fire hydrant" method of information giving, providing an abundance of information that could, inadvertently, overwhelm the recipient and discourage additional questions or conversational depth.

(Continued)

Table 14.2 (Continued)

Specific Suggestions	A sex therapist may prescribe an activity or "homework" for the client with the goal of improving sexual satisfaction, not unlike a temporary agreement (depending on how it is delivered).
Intensive Therapy	This would be a recommendation of individual therapy, group therapy, and/or medication management for any of the system members presenting for sex therapy. Such would focus on decreasing individual distress and potentially diving deeper into their history and intrapersonal stressors, such as past trauma.

We could also add an "EX" at the beginning to give someone time to "Ex"-press their thoughts, feelings, current perceptions, and misgivings related to sexuality as a whole. You could say, to learn more about the person's context!

Sensate-Focused Therapy

Sensate-focused therapy could be considered a form of physical touch exposure therapy in the specific context of one's relationship. It is more behaviorally focused than PLISSIT and, in some ways, could be a gradual example of the "specific suggestions" step. It includes five levels over two stages, sensual and sexual:

1. First is *non-demand physical touch*, forbidding sexual intercourse during this phase. The purpose of this limitation is to help the person struggling with touch to not feel pressured and decrease the linear alignment of sensual touch as foreplay, allowing it to be an intimate act by itself. At this level, participants take turns touching the other as they want to be touched on parts of the body not overtly affiliated with sex; both parties can notice what they like or dislike, and eventually the recipient can request specific changes to pressure or guide the giver's movements.
2. The second level expands on the process of the first, now including (though not limited to) *touch to non-genital sexualized body parts* such as the chest and thighs. Turning the recipient on is not the goal. Instead, it is to build a sense of safety and to know the touch is a bridge of intimacy, not a demand for more. The recipient can provide feedback to what feels good and what body parts they realize are sensual for them specifically (ears, feet, wrists, collar line, and so on).
3. The third level adds *genitalia touch* to the experience, primarily *for the purpose of learning to be comfortable* with this physical part of

your own and your partner's body, growing in safety with one another. Arousing the recipient still is not the goal.

4. At the fourth level, if someone with a vagina is part of the dynamic, the giver may practice *insertion without movement*, practicing self- and partner-soothing. For those with a penis, this could also include insertion of an orifice or gripping the phallus. Some duos choose to skip this step.

5. The final level is *non-demand intercourse*, meaning the goal is pleasure, not orgasm. As with before, the purpose is tied to mindful awareness of the present and one's body and comfort within the moment.

A systemic version of this therapy would emphasize the roles, assumptions, communication, and pleasure of both partners throughout each level. These are the therapeutic values that most closely resemble CRT.

Sexual Assessment Questions

There are specific questions or versions of questions for CRT sex therapy. These aim to openly guide clients to reflect on their histories, definitions, and meaning-making of sexual concepts and experiences. Learning these histories about partners also helps alleviate resentment or personalization with a partner through compassionate contextualization. We better understand how they came to their beliefs or why parts of them struggle with current dynamics. We will later use this in circular questions ("*What happens for you when you hear your partner describe this past experience?*")

Here are some CRT sex therapy assessment questions:

1. "*Where and how did you learn about sex? Who were your primary 'teachers'? If you wanted to know something that your teacher wouldn't teach you, how did you learn it?*"
2. "*What emotions are associated with the topic of sex? How about the act of sex?*"
3. "*How would you describe yourself as a sexual person? What words come to mind?*" (Examples: spontaneous, giving, explorative, passionate, naive, uncomfortable)
4. "*What comes to mind or heart when you hear me ask about pleasure? Fantasy? Solo play? Monogamy?*"

We can also use scaling questions to learn about current sexual or intimacy perceptions and the clients' goals:

5. "*On a scale of 1 to 10, how satisfied are you with your current sex life, 1 being completely unsatisfied, and 10 being completely satisfied and fulfilled?*"

6. *"On a scale of 1 to 10, how connected do you feel with your sexual partner(s), 1 being completely detached and disconnected emotionally, and 10 being completely satisfied and fulfilled? How connected do you want to be?"*
7. *"On a scale of 1 to 10, how aware are you of your sexual preferences, such as what you find sexy, desirable, or arousing? 1 being completely unaware or uncomfortable at the idea of learning these about yourself, and 10 being capable and willing of providing a list of attributes?"*

As always, even in early sessions that are assessment-focused, we can apply interventions, such as clarifying definitions and meaning-making and compassionate contextualization.

CRT Intervention Applications

In this section, we highlight a few different CRT intervention applications pertaining to sex therapy, which may also be expanded on in the next two chapters.

Intentional Language

In CRT, meaning-making comes directly from language intentionality: exploring and cultivating a deep understanding of what the words, ideas, and experiences mean. All too often in relationships, one person has a definition of what something means that is different from what their partner has. We saw this with our case study in Chapter 13, where what one person defined as cheating was different from what their partner defined as cheating. Remember two ground rules for meaning-making: (1) the client sets the original meaning, and the therapist can reframe it as helpful; and (2) compassionately disentangling past meaning from current identity is central to sexual identity congruence and sex therapy outcomes. Here are a few commonly used terms and ideas where meaning-making of language can be clarified:

- Intimacy
- Nakedness
- Having sex versus intercourse versus making love versus fucking
- Identifying as "sexually active"
- High versus low sex drive
- Spontaneity, adventurousness, or being experimental
- Eroticism, desire, or pleasure
- Erotic or non-erotic touch

More specific terms may come up for specific clients that will also be worth clarifying as we go.

Positive Memory Restoration

It is common for sex therapy to also include interventions that build emotional intimacy, often looking similar to couples therapy. Therefore, we will also apply relational reflections pertaining to sex:

o "When was a time this week you felt *connected with or cared for by* your partner?"
o "When was a time this week that you felt *drawn or attracted to* your partner?"
o "When was a time this week that you saw your partner needed *intimate connection*?"
o "When was a time this week that you *felt sexy*? How did you let your partner know? How did they respond? How did that response feel for you?"
o "What is something you hope your partner knows about *your sexual availability* going into this next week?"

Reflecting on past intimate compassionate connections within a sexual dynamic can help strengthen the bond.

Temporary Agreements

Temporary agreements pertaining to sex can be as straightforward as trying a new sexual position or practicing asking questions overtly around interests or curiosities. As previously mentioned, participating in sensate-focused therapy, or variations of it, could be considered a type of temporary agreement. For example, for those who find it hard to find time and energy for sex, or where context switching (jumping from one thing to the other spontaneously) is challenging, create a temporary agreement to schedule sex into the week.

Agree to try a day and time for sex to be on the schedule, set rules and parameters around how to approach it, and agree to try it for one week with the opportunity for re-evaluation the next time you're in therapy. As much as possible, let's encourage clients to have fun and be silly in these agreements to reiterate the purpose is connection and enjoyment, not a checklist of "have we tried this yet?"

Modality Comparison: Solution-Focused Therapy (SFT)

Unlike PLISSIT or senate-focused therapy, solution-focused therapy (SFT) is not specific to sex therapy. This is also true of CRT. In SFT, questions focus on strengths of the client system and what has worked for them in the past, even just a little bit or for a little while. In SFT, the therapist may work with the client to draw parallels from one situation to another in the client's life, such as how they speak their needs in one context versus another. As identified in Chapter 4, SFT is defined by the types of questions it asks, which can be summarized into three types: desired possible outcomes, exception-seeking, and scaling questions.

In sex therapy, this would be talking about what the pairing's intimate relationship would look like if the problem of sex was not there – How would they interact differently? How would their sex be different? If these are their goals for treatment, what would they see in themselves and one another that tells them they are working toward those? How have they worked through relational hardships before? What have they already tried, and did some small piece of that work that we can expand on?

Though not framed in the same way, CRT also aims to focus on parts of life that can be changed – what can we control versus what we cannot – and the small steps it takes to get there. We are also strengths based in the intentional exploration and fostering of what the client does well ("Do more of what works"), not letting persistent problems overshadow these.

A few key differences between SFT and CRT with sex therapy is the intentional exploration beyond behavioral change, addressing shame potentially tied to the subject. CRT also is not exclusively focused on the present and future like SFT; we must acknowledge and give compassion to how past experiences inform the present – context! This includes our past sexual selves and the building of intimate and sexual safety with a partner through compassion as a foundation to express one authentic sexual self, which SFT does not address directly.

Case Study

Let's look at a new relationship for this section of the book. Daniel is a 29-year-old Caucasian heterosexual man. He and his wife, 28-year-old Sylvia, who identifies as Hispanic, have been together for just under a year. Both hold full-time jobs – Daniel works as an accountant while Sylvia works as a social media manager – and have been living together for the past four months to save on bills. As you work your way through the first few intake sessions, you figure out that the couple is experiencing frequent arguments and "challenges" with sex and intimacy. The couple explains that they're not on the "same page" when it comes to sex and that they "both want different things." They report feeling frustrated and disappointed that this part of their relationship feels so challenging. In the session we're looking at, we're exploring one area of the sexual relationship that is challenging for the couple – the different sex drives they have.

Therapist: Okay y'all, so it seems like one of the challenges we're navigating is that you both feel as though your sex drive looks different than your partner's. I'd love for each of you to tell me a little bit more about what you feel like this sex drive looks like for you. (*Disentangling meaning-making*)

Daniel: I feel like we just have such different ideas of what a "high sex drive" looks like. I don't know. I feel like we have sex maybe once a week on average, and I honestly feel satisfied with that. I also don't feel like I need to have sex any more than that.

Sylvia: Ugh, I get so disheartened when I hear that. It makes me feel like there's something wrong with me because I want a more active sex life than that. For me, when I think of a high sex drive I think of people who are fucking like every single day. I know for me, I'd be totally open to something like that, but feel like Daniel can't meet me there.

T: Okay, thanks for cueing me into what that idea looks like for the two of you. It seems as though we have some different perspectives on what a "high sex drive" looks like, and what we would want sex to look like in the relationship as well.

D: Yeah, I think it just became clear to me how fundamentally different some of our perspectives are, like our whole schemas are just opposite.

S: We really do. There's so much frustration for me that comes up when I would hear you talking about having a high sex drive and that we have a high level of sexual activity in the relationship because it didn't resonate with me at all. I feel so differently and now I'm realizing, oh literally we have completely different definitions of what that means. It's like we're looking at two completely different shades of blue, one that's super light and the other completely dark and claiming them both as blue.

T: Absolutely, and let me tell you what I love about this. We're really seeing that for the two of you, there seems to be a lot of distress stemming from a lack of understanding of your partner's definitions and expectations of what something means. "I'm curious, what difference does it make to shift this perspective, or consider other possibilities?" (*Meaning-making disentangling/nonjudg-mental curiosity/multipartiality*)

S: Well, it makes me feel like I'm not crazy for one. I felt like we were so incompatible and couldn't communicate and now I realize that we weren't speaking the same language and this felt like a translation that cleared some things up.

D: Yeah, I feel like it helps me to know where Sylvia's at. I felt really judged for not feeling similarly and like I wasn't meeting her needs, and I see now that from her perspective I actually haven't been. (*perpetual opportunity for compassion*).

S: I'm glad that it feels like he can understand why this has felt so challenging for me. I think I wonder though, like yeah it's great that we can see these new perspectives, but I don't know how to get my needs met, because I don't want to have to compromise my sexual experience and drive just because my partner's drive is different. Unless there's something wrong with that and I should just learn to be okay with what Daniel wants?

T: I'm really glad you're bringing that up, that's a huge part of this as well. Just because Daniel's sex drive might look different than yours doesn't mean that we want you to compromise your sexual experience either. *(psychoeducation addressing misinformation)* I want us to continue exploring this idea and exploring what it would look like for you both to have your sexual needs authentically met in the relationship.

Chapter 15

Compassionately Removing Sexual Judgments

Have you ever heard yourself or someone else start a sentence with, "Okay, don't judge me, but. . ."? It's usually followed up by a statement or story that we judge ourselves for. Even in therapy, which is hypothetically our "safe space," we hear clients say this, almost like a confessional, seeking acceptance but doubting its viability. On a day-to-day basis, many of us fear that we're going to be judged for how we look, what we wear, what we eat or drink, what we buy, how we communicate . . . literally any choice we make. We change our appearance, behaviors, and even how we talk to try and avoid the judgmental, condescending, and hurtful glare or side eye. And it makes sense! Judgment is tied to rejection; it is a survival response to not want to be rejected. We recognize this is a pattern in life and relationships as a whole.

> **A Note from Emma:** Moment of honesty. Let's be real. We've all had a moment of being judgmental toward someone – a stranger, a colleague, or a loved one – at some point or situation. It's human and it's ingrained early on in life. Let's also call it for what it can be – harmful, painful, and destructive (both to ourselves and another). However, we also know there is much more to us than those actions. We acknowledge our actions for what they are/were and work to repair any rupture that has occurred from them.

Sexual expression and interaction can already feel at times vulnerable, raw, and exposing. Sex and sensuality introduces new spaces to fear judgment: for your body, the size or appearance of certain body parts, how your body moves, how you orgasm, for your interests or what relaxes you sexually, or how you talk flirty or dirty. And we fear these judgments not only for current thoughts or behaviors; maybe you've been or felt judged for your sexual past. Judgment can feel so isolating, whether from others or from ourselves.

DOI: 10.4324/9781003518730-19

Let's be real, this is something we all experience, both as the judged or judger. If that's you, welcome to the club; you're human. There's no shame in that. This chapter will focus on how we use the concepts of CRT to intentionally decrease sexual judgment or discomfort to create space for nonjudgmental curiosity in ourselves and sexual relationships.

Nonjudgmental Sexual Curiosity

A lot of people have different perceptions on why we judge ourselves and others: Maybe we do it for status and self-righteous social comparison, to boost confidence, to assuage our inner critique, or maybe because we're just terrible people who should know better (well, that sounds judgmental . . .). In this context, judgment is more than comparison; it is an appraisal of acceptability. While comparison can be a feature of this (and once again the influence of technology and media in the judgment game cannot be underestimated here), it is the damnation of the unexpected or unaccepted. Who determines what is accepted? Usually it's the most dominant narrative – not because it is correct, but because it is the loudest. And as said earlier, when survival is dependent on fitting in, we lose motivation to announce what makes us unique. So we buy into the social assumption that behaviors, thoughts, interests, tastes, and methods outside that norm are deviant, faulty, or even something to feel ashamed of. This is where we hear, "What's wrong with me; why am I like this?"

And this is the hypothetical question we get to answer: Why are we like this? Not only about sexual interests but about meta- and chronosystems with a fixation on sexuality and, more specifically, controlling narratives around sexuality:

- *"When are some of the early experiences you remember being judged? Being judgmental?"*
- *"When was an early memory of someone else commenting on your body?"*
- *"Where did you learn that specific interest was unacceptable?"*

These questions are appropriate for both the revealing curious individual and their audience, such as a partner. As clients identify this context to engrained sexual judgments, CRT therapists can intentionally lean into questions rooted in curiosity and shared excitement for the client's authenticity:

- *"I'm so honored you let me know about that! What is it like to tell someone and have them receive it with encouragement and excitement?"*
- *"How did you learn you like/dislike that? What is it like to let yourself have that preference without making it a big deal or shrinking it down to insignificance?"*

- *"What is it like to be reminded that sexual pleasure is frequently self-taught for people?"*
- *"How does it feel to hear that you are not even the only client I have/have had with that curiosity?"*

Having the therapist establish this acceptance without hesitation early in sex-focused conversations is akin to unconditional positive regard in sexual conversations. If there are others present, such as a partner, we must also include them in the conversation.

This helps avoid the perception of one person being the focus/problem in therapy – multipartiality! – and creates a space where both can ask questions about past and current interactions, hopes, and comfortability without either partner being "the problem" for how they receive or give this information. I've heard in sessions before when a client said, "I only did that because I thought you liked that," or "I had no idea that's something you wanted." Therapy can be where partners, even for the first time, talk about experiences and preferences and really get to know about each other as whole sexual beings. While we are talking about this with tones of excitement – that's our biases coming out – we recognize not everyone feels this way about sex, let alone niche sexual interests.

Especially in the face of niche sexual interests, or new spaces of exploration for couples, it can be helpful to explore where on a scale of "no interest" to "very interested," they would land with certain sexual activities. This scale would move from levels of "no interest," to "minimal interest but open," to "mildly curious to try," and winding up at "very interested to try." We can also ask if the act or kink we're talking about is something that's been tried before, or something that sounds appealing in an effort to create open dialogue and dispel shaming. When it comes to CRT, this would fall under the category of disentangling (i.e. meaning making, assumption of intent), as we're working to understand perspective, assumption, and how things have occurred.

Nonjudgmental Sexual Flavors: Vanilla is Delicious

A Note from Bethany: One of my favorite metaphors about sex is ice cream. There are many flavors and toppings, countless combinations and preferences, and so much exploring that can happen! Best of all, they can both be amazing! Of course, there is always something to be said for a bowl of vanilla ice cream. It's not boring when it's exactly what I want. For more information about this, check out Stefani Goerlich's book, *With Sprinkles on Top*.

In the years the authors have been practicing therapy, we've both seen an uptick in couples who show up in the therapy space wanting to "spice up" a "vanilla" relationship. They come in and announce that they have a "boring" sex life and that things aren't "spontaneous," "new," or "fun" anymore. Oftentimes, we see it where one person may want to introduce different sexual elements, and the other doesn't feel quite as comfortable with it, or doesn't even know about it. When people talk about their vanilla relationships or sex lives, there are a few assumptions to dismantle:

1. Everyone's definition of "vanilla" is different the same (Can't be! Hello, meaning-making and disentangling!)
2. "Vanilla" is bad, boring, or inadequate sex.
3. The threshold for sexual experimentation and freedom seems to be getting more lofty. Once you add a metaphorical topping, or try something new, that does not have to become the new standard or norm. This is the cornerstone of CRT temporary agreements.

Unfortunately, people can be judgmental toward vanilla sex just as much as any other flavor. So let's set the message clearly: Vanilla is not bad. Vanilla is not plain. It is a flavor that can have variety, depth, and add deliciousness to whatever it spices. Everyone deserves to enjoy what you like confidently! Vanilla is simply another sexual style and way of presenting in a relationship, one often associated with coziness and security, which is hardly something to judge.

We can learn about client perceptions of vanilla, both relationally and sexually, through meaning-making questions:

1. What does a vanilla sexual and intimate life look like and feel like for you?
2. When you think of a vanilla relationship, what comes to mind?
3. What are your needs in a sexual and intimate relationship?

All this ties back into our sexual and personal values, attitudes, and behaviors striving for congruence with one another. As we pursue that authenticity for our clients, we also want to avoid over-personalizing assumptions, such as what it means to enjoy versus *be* "vanilla." Destigmatization via disentangling is needed to cultivate relational compassion. CRT approaches this through *"and"* language that honors and appreciates current relationship strengths amidst potential new flavor tastings.

When Judgment Presents as Disgust

If we're going to be talking about judgment, we also have to talk about disgust, because sometimes disgust frankly feels unavoidable. One of the topics that has most resonated with the authors throughout their sex therapy training (and personal work) is the concept of *sexual disgust*, or feelings of distaste or discomfort pertaining to sexuality, including the experiences and preferences of self or others, physical features or organs, or sexual thoughts. Sexual disgust frequently results in sexual aversion or avoidance.

Look, disgust is the ick. Take a moment and think about something that disgusts you. Maybe it is a certain sensory sensation, like a smell or taste? Maybe an experience you had or witnessed? Maybe it's a word, like moist, suckled, or pus (Did anyone else just gag a little?). Notice what comes up for you with this. What does disgust feel like in your body? Identifying disgust and how it shows up is helpful for when we encounter a sexual situation that induces that same feeling in us. This is sexual mindfulness.

Sexually, disgust can surface when we think about past partners, interactions, settings, and the like. Here are just a few client quotes that convey some of the variety of ways sexual disgust can show up:

o "*I can't believe* I slept with them."
o "How is cum both sticky and slick? *It's gross.*"
o "I didn't know women had vaginal discharge besides periods. *Ew.*"
o "*I can't imagine* someone actually finding me attractive."
o "I found nudes my partner received from someone else; *that is disgusting.*"
o "*Can you believe* my partner masturbates to videos of tattooed women on the internet? *Is that normal?*"
o "Did you hear she got pregnant? *What a waste.*"
o "You had sex *there?*"
o "When I saw his penis, *I wanted to just get up and run.*"
o "They reached over and put their hand on my leg, and I felt like *I wanted to vomit.*"

We know that disgust can be in close proximity to shame, envy, contempt, and hurt. When disgust shows up, oftentimes those other emotions follow. These examples all show language of judgement overlapped with disgust, and there are many ways that can look. What can feel sexually disgusting to one person might not feel sexually disgusting to another.

One of the most common occurrences for sexual disgust is conversations about past sexuality. In CRT, we believe that clients are the experts in their own lives. They are also the keepers of their own context and meaning-making. Both in broad strokes or specific questions, CRT therapists ask how past events contribute to approaches in communication, sex, and roles in relationships and use this information to stay present and future focused: *"How does learning this information feel beneficial?"*

As always, the goal is not to judge the disgusted part of a person. Oftentimes, when people experience sexual disgust, they feel like they're wrong for feeling it and should be a "more accepting person." Treating those around us with acceptance and kindness is essential, *and* the disgust has context, not the person. If one person feels like the source of the disgust, the therapist may intervene to identify the disgust as a rigid part that may lack self-compassion for their own deviations from social norms, sexually or otherwise. The therapist can exemplify to clients' loved ones how to rephrase inquiries with curiosity, not judgment (see Table 15.1).

You may notice these questions are very cognitive and not as emotion-based. We want to also hold space for emotions; sometimes it can be a surprise to hear a loved one, particularly an intimate partner, has withheld a part of them. However, in a moment of vulnerable authenticity, we want the attention to stay on the sharing partner to give them space to receive the partner's compassionate nonjudgment. If the partner appears unable or unwilling to do this in session, we can slow down to have the therapist validate each person, starting with the sharing partner, until each partner is more regulated and feels "heard" by the therapist first before trying compassionate contextualization again. Comparable to sex, we do

Table 15.1 Nonjudgmental Curiosity Questions about Sexuality

Try this. . .	*. . . instead of these*
"I'm struggling to understand. What contributed to this situation occurring?"	"How could you find yourself in that position if you said you didn't want to do that?"
"Can I ask what about that activity feels connecting and appealing for you?"	"Why would you like that?"
"I don't remember hearing about this before. Will you tell me more or clarify that detail?"	"Why wouldn't you tell me about that?"
"I'm trying to understand this. Can you explain a little more what led up to this?"	"Why would you do something like that?"
"I haven't experienced this before. How do you hope or envision this being part of this relationship?"	"That's so weird you like that; I just don't get it."

not want to breeze past the disgusted part; we want its consent to move the conversation forward, too.

When Judgment Presents as Comparison

One of the biggest fears associated with the past is our friend, comparison. Comparison creates a means to quantify, and if it remains that non-judgmental, it isn't bad. From a therapeutic perspective, we can explore/quantify what has worked, not worked, or worked a little bit or for a little while. This is different from pinning people or experiences against each other. There is a huge difference between saying, "Here's something that I know feels good for me," versus, "You're not as good at that as my vibrator," or, "You're not as open minded as my ex." This is where we see a shift from comparison to judgment. It leaves little room for naivety or curiosity. Instead, CRT seeks to ask and answer, *"What if this isn't as insurmountably problematic as we are treating it?"* If comparison is something you're noticing within yourself, exploring where it's coming from, and why it's showing up can help us understand some of our responses, nervousness, or insecurity. Furthermore, when we're experiencing insecurity as a result of inner comparison, exploring with a partner or partners what our needs might be surrounding affirmation, or encouragement could also be beneficial.

Compassionately Communicating Kinks and Fetishes

If there was a sexual spectrum with vanilla on one end, people often assume kink is at the other end. However, we propose that kink is the spectrum itself! Fetishes fall onto that spectrum. Kinks come in all shapes, sizes, and varieties. As clinicians, we have learned there is always another kink out there that we haven't heard about. With the rise of media and technology, access to kink material and community has never been easier. We also know that being on either end of the kink spectrum – vanilla or highly socially stigmatized – there is often a lot of judgment in how someone experiences sexual pleasure. Even within the kink community, there is sometimes more acceptance for certain types of kinks or fetishes than others. In relationships, navigating kink preferences, experience, and comfort can be a challenge, especially if the topic has drastically different meaning-making to each person.

There can be a lot of fear and nervousness surrounding sharing a kink preference with a partner; there can be surprisingly similar emotions when hearing about a partner's kink interests. This can be especially true if these drastically differ from the sexual norms so far. In both cases, the possibility of this being a threat to the relationship looms.

First, we want to say that compassion goes both ways. There needs to be compassion for the partner desiring or expressing the kink, while also needing to be compassion for the partner receiving this information. Sometimes a partner can feel surprised or confused initially when hearing about a kink or preference. Naturally, this can feel judgmental. While we embrace the spectrum of sexual engagement and preferences, we also recognize that everyone's experience, exposure, and comfort with kink varies. Both the kink and the response make sense in context.

Introducing Kink and Fetish into a Relationship

Once the specific sexual interest is identified, we can use *temporary agreements* in kink exploration. This is our intervention application for this chapter.

Especially when thinking about introducing a new relationship dynamic or activity, the purpose of temporary is tied to mindfulness.

In session, participants can agree to a set time frame (a week, a month, etc.) to try an introductory level of the kink. They get to decide what that looks like. While participating and immediately after, participants are encouraged to privately reflect on it:

- How does my body feel during the kink participation? What physically feels good or bad about this?
- What feels connecting or disconnecting?
- What thoughts or emotions did this bring up in me?
- What questions did this bring up in me?

Participants can decide whether or not to share that independently or in the next therapy session.

Alternatively, the partners may temporarily agree to *not* participate in the kink for a month and review the same questions about that sexual experience. It is common to do a temporary agreement each way, one after another. The participants get full say on the boundaries and parameters of the temporary agreements. Finding new, fun, and spicy ways to lean into agreements can still allow for some creativity, while also pacing things out in a way that works for them.

In our work as CRT therapists, part of our role is to distinguish kink understanding or acceptance versus partner acceptance as a person. When working to communicate about kinks, we always want to explore (A) Is this something the partner is able or interested in doing, and (B) Is this a part of their partner that they can accept? We need to understand if it is positive or aversive for the other partner. Oftentimes in relationships, people will either:

- Accept the kink as part of person and relationship, fully participating in it together
- Accept the kink as part of person and relationship, conditionally participating in it together
- Accept the kink as part of person and not the relationship, creating alternative methods to meet the desire for the kink to be met
- Accept the kink as part of a person and not the relationship, resulting in the kink being absent overall.
- Not accept the kink as part of a person or the relationship, potentially leading to the dissolution of the relationship.

As CRT therapists, we don't push any particular option onto the couples. Instead, we work to empower them to make the decision and choice that works best for them and the relationship. As always, safety and trust are both the means and the goal of communicating around kinks. We want all individuals involved to feel comfortable and supported without judgment. This can frequently be achieved through temporary agreements.

Modality Comparison: Accelerated Experiential Dynamic Psychotherapy (AEDP)

One of the newer therapy modalities from the last decades is Accelerated Experiential Dynamic Psychotherapy (AEDP), coined and created by Dr. Diana Fosha. AEDP cultivates client change through providing a relational experience with their therapist that mobilizes positive change via increased neuroplasticity in the brain. AEDP believes in the fundamental power that not feeling alone in an experience or emotion can help us process through them. Within sex therapy, AEDP believes that the restorative relationship between client and therapist, while also focusing on the "here and now" of emotions can help facilitate decreased dependence on sexual behaviors that feel distressing for clients. They also believe that AEDO can help heal attachment wounds that lead to clients engaging in sexual behaviors that they find distressing. This ties into one of the main commonalities between AEDP and CRT. Both of these modalities believe and prioritize the relationship with the therapist, *and* the therapist provides a relationship that alleviates loneliness. One main difference is that AEDP focuses more on the healing of trauma versus all experiences that the client would want to process. There can be an emphasis on changing previous defensive tactics used to avoid/cope with trauma, and instead search for parts of the client that are "underused" or "untapped resources." AEDP will focus on increasing the use of those parts of the client, increasing awareness of innate client coping skills that were "always there."

Case Study

Let's return to Daniel and Sylvia. They've continued to show up routinely to sessions and are committed to trying to create change in the relationship. You've discovered that one part of their sexual relationship that experiences challenges is in their respective sexual styles and personalities.

T:	Okay, Sylvia, I remember you expressing that the way you and Dan engage sexually can feel like an area of challenge for you. Can you tell me a little bit more about what you mean by that?
S:	Yeah, I just feel like Dan is really different than anyone I've ever been with before. Like when it comes to sex I'm used to guys who really make it known that they want me and who are more dominant. I don't know how to interact with someone like that.
T:	Hmm, okay Sylvia, I want to make sure I'm understanding you correctly, what I'm hearing is that Dan's sexual personality is one that's new to you, and it seems like you're working to get more familiar with what that looks like in the relationship.
S:	Yeah, I mean it's just so like foreign to me to have a guy sexually interact with me with such low levels of intensity and like passion. I don't know, I mean it's good that he doesn't like to hurt me or do really intense things, but it's just so gentle and soft all the time.
T:	Okay, I hear that Sylvia. If it's okay, I'm going to hear a bit from Dan on his thoughts. Dan, what's coming up for you as we talk about this?
D:	Uh, yeah, I feel like who I am sexually isn't good enough or acceptable. Like the fact that I'm not this crazy intense dominant guy isn't okay and I have to be that way to sexually satisfy. I'd also say that I don't agree that I'm not passionate or intense, because I feel like I am those things.

T:	Thank you for that Dan, that makes a lot of sense to me. I wonder if some of what we're experiencing is different definitions of what "passionate" or "intense" look like. *(Disentangling-meaning making)*
D:	I also feel like Sylvia is judging me for who I am which makes me want to withdraw even more.
T:	It seems like you feel a bit hurt by that Dan.
D:	Yeah, hurt and frustrated.
S:	I'm not trying to judge him, it's more that I just don't know how to handle it and I also know what I find attractive and like a lot of what I would define as gentleness isn't super erotic to me.
T:	I hear that Sylvia. Your erotic needs are valued and feeling interacted with sexually in the way that you enjoy is important. I'm curious, Dan, what about interacting with Sylvia in the ways that you do feel connecting and appealing? *(non-judgmental sexual curiosity)*
D:	It makes me feel like I'm really treasuring her and savoring the experience with her to go slowly and move gently. I want her to feel beautiful and valued and moving through things aggressively and quickly doesn't feel like I'm doing that for her.
T:	That's a really beautiful way to phrase that Dan, I hear your intention there and your desire to make Sylvia feel as valued as possible.
S:	I appreciate that he wants me to feel valued and treasured, that means a lot for me to hear. I also know that even if that's his intention, rough sex communicates and means something different for me than it does for him.
T:	That makes sense Sylvia. So, I'm going to ask you the same question, what about rough sex feels appealing and connecting for you? *(non-judgmental sexual curiosity reciprocated)*
S:	It makes me feel desired and wanted. And feeling that way boosts my confidence both sexually and in the other areas of relationship as well.

Chapter 16

Trauma, Sexuality, and CRT

As a therapist, counselor, or educator, working with traumatized individuals is inevitable. There are many forms of trauma – addiction, hate crimes, poverty, neglect, and abuse of all kinds. This chapter will specifically look at the impact of trauma on a person's authentic self-expression, particularly sexually. That being said, we don't want to get stuck in content. Regardless of the trauma source, compassionate relational approaches can remain consistent.

Defining Trauma

There have been many definitions of trauma as we come to better understand it. Bessel Van der Kolk, author of *The Body Keeps the Score*, says trauma is not the past events but the imprint they leave on the mind and soul. The prolonging of pain is what causes suffering, not the pain itself. This is why trauma can be so subjective and what traumatizes one person may not traumatize someone else. Dan Allender, founder of the Allender Center of trauma treatment, defines it relationally as the overt absence of care in the face of harm or terror or a sense of powerlessness and helplessness in a current circumstance. All this speaks to the innately relational nature of trauma. People have a relationship with their memories, and the relationship can be traumatic. Those memories can include events, people, dates, sensory cues, and many other attributes.

Sources of Trauma

Based on existing research, CRT classifies trauma in language of relational wounds. These are present at all levels of co-occurring systems, immediate self and beyond:

1. Abandonment – sense of emotional or physical loss (such as grief), or being left
2. Betrayal – trust given and broken

DOI: 10.4324/9781003518730-20

3. Humiliation – embarrassment or public degradation
4. Injustice – criticism or rigid punitive action, emotional indifference/distance
5. Rejection – not being chosen, being seen but discarded

Any of these can be experienced directly or secondarily. Secondary trauma occurs when a person's empathic hearing of someone else's story is difficult to distinguish from their own pain (remember enmeshment?), resulting in comparable symptoms of the painful event happening to them directly. When this happens repeatedly, it can be called vicarious trauma, which shifts a person's worldview based on repeated exposure to traumatic events.

Trauma can also stem from wider systemic or collective experiences, particularly the psychological reaction to significant macro- or chronosystemic events, such as:

• COVID-19
• Lasting impacts of racism, past and present
• Religious trauma
• Indigenous trauma

> **A Note from Bethany:** I've heard some people complain, "Everyone says they have trauma nowadays!" To this I say. . . you're right! The mental health industry broadened the definition of trauma, recognizing how extensively past events impact people. Trauma is the result of when a stressor surpasses one's coping capacities. The historically used "Suck it up, Buttercup" attitude requires emotional suppression, which is different from emotional regulation. Regulation is more closely tied to resilience and compassion.

Trauma Rooted in Abuse and Neglect

Though categorized in numerous ways, abuse and neglect can fall into six groups:

○ Physical
○ Sexual
○ Verbal/Emotional
○ Psychological/Mental
○ Financial
○ Identity/Cultural

These cover specific sources such as medical, technological, domestic, discriminatory, and institutional abuse and neglect. Key attributes of abuse and neglect are the absence or revoking of consent and a strict hierarchical split that is restrictive and harmful to the person(s) not in positions of power. Abusive behaviors can be aggressive physical contact; harassment; intimidation; insults; coercion; manipulation; fraud; lack of privacy; and restricting resources, material and nonmaterial, such as education. Bear in mind, abuse and neglect can be harm from others or ourselves via shame, contempt, or ambivalence toward our own wellbeing. Abuse occurs across all ages, ethnicities and races, socioeconomic state, religious affiliations, and roles. However, minorities and those at other social disadvantages are consistently at a higher risk.

Sexual abuse, in particular, impacts sexual relationships and self-expression. Specific forms are:

- Sexual assault (nonconsensual participation in or observation of sexual activities)
- Sexual harassment (unwillingly receiving gender-based stereotyping or sexually suggestive messages, verbally or behaviorally);
- Stalking
- Intimate partner violence/control (IPV)

According to data from the USA Centers for Injury Prevention and Control, Division of Violence Prevention, approximately 44% of women (52.2 million) and 25% of men (27.6 million) reported experiencing contact sexual violence at some time in their life. The most common perpetrators of sexual abuse are current or former intimate partners. Though not exclusionary, sexual abuse is most prevalent in women ages 16–24 and impacts approximately 25–40% of families in the USA. Worldwide, numbers range for 8–31% of girls and 3–17% of boys experience childhood sexual abuse. Child physical abuse, maltreatment, and neglect were more prevalent among individuals who also experience sexual abuse than those without. The frequency, type, and number of sexual abuse encounters bears significant positive correlation with psychopathology. In total, it is easy to see how deeply trauma integrates into sexual wellbeing.

Trauma Rooted in Religious Experiences

Religious trauma is the psychological result of pain brought on by religious messages, beliefs, and experiences. This frequently occurs over prolonged exposure rather than acute events, potentially prompted by poignant interactions and quotes from significant figures in the organization. It differs from spiritual abuse in its degree of subjectivity and thematic presences, whereas spiritual abuse is more overtly harmful or abusive interactions with religiously affiliated individual(s), often in positions of influence/leadership. Of course, they are not necessarily mutually exclusive, such as conversion or reparative therapies. Research endorses abundant evidence that religious organizations and doctrine have been harmful, controlling, and judgmental, particularly among sexual identities beyond cis/heterosexuality.

Symptoms of Trauma

Relational traumas innately turn inward to create intrapersonal distress, manifesting in symptoms of intrusive thoughts, personalization, hyperarousal, hypervigilance, perfectionism, physiological distress such as gastrointestinal problems, numbness, dissociation, compulsion to reenact, restriction of range of affect, and sleep disturbances. In relationships, trauma contributes to increased difficulty trusting others or setting or holding boundaries. Religious trauma, specifically, perpetuates dispositional shame and discourages critical thinking. The latter is a common result of hermeneutical injustice, when oppressive social systems restrict access to knowledge in order to diminish personal agency and maintain existing power hierarchies.

All forms of trauma can greatly impact a person's mental, sexual, and relational health. Sexual and religious trauma, in particular, can impact sexual functioning. This may manifest as misconceptions about consent, physiological sexual dysfunction, sexually related phobias, distress receiving medical care, and anxiety and depressive symptoms including suicidality. Looking specifically at trauma's impact on gender and sexuality, there are numerous impacts to potentially disentangle:

- Misperceptions about sexual activity as primarily focused on reproduction or obligation, not pleasure. Even after marriage, non-vanilla sex can still be viewed as deviant.
- Fixation on concepts of "purity," especially in females. Includes misinformation regarding measures of uterine virginity, like the intact hymen.
- Detering independent sexual exploration and treating education as innately lustful.
- Misperceptions of individual responsibility, such as women responsible for the men who lust after them.
- Internalized homo- and transphobia.
- Internalized assumptions of the necessity of a lifelong partner (singular) and what a "normal" sex drive is, neglecting the very normal experiences of asexuality and/or aromanticism.
- Difficulty transitioning the view of sex from threatening/problematic to safe/connecting.

- Understanding of gender constructs – utilizing the binary and corresponding sociologically assigned behaviors with biological sex to "gender train" someone in how to be a boy or girl and assess ability/willingness to adhering to those limits.
- Bodily discomfort tied to chronic shame – based on the Pentateuch's message regarding original sin, correlating nudity and shame.
- Affiliating self-worth with maintaining sexual abstinence.

There can also be a significant physiological impact and prominence of sexual functionality issues in all four classes of sexual disorders (see Table 16.1).

Unfortunately, like other forms of trauma, physical and emotional distance from the trauma's source does not necessarily end the associated symptoms. The hurt and the healing is in the relationship with the pain, not the pain itself.

Table 16.1 Sexual Disorder Classifications

Diagnostic Class	Sexual Disorders
Desire	Low libido
Arousal	Erectile disorder, female sexual arousal disorder, premature ejaculation
Orgasm	Delayed ejaculation, female orgasmic disorder
Pain	Genito-pelvic pain/penetration disorders

CRT Perspective on Trauma

As stated earlier, CRT approaches trauma not as a part of one's past but the relationship with parts of our past. We can have a traumatic relationship with past, current, or possible future events. Change in that relationship, increasing compassion for that past version of ourselves and other system members, can decrease traumatic symptomology.

To quote a recent training by Dr. Bornell Nicholson, "The line between our trauma and our goodness is thin." Our positive attributes can be used against us in traumatic situations, including our kindness, diligence, reliability, honesty, thoughtfulness, open-mindedness, sense of fairness, and respect for others, among others. CRT reclaims these as strengths, folding them into existing qualities of resilience. We approach the pain source with the same lens of curiosity and nonjudgment as other presenting problems. The clinician is responsible to consistently assess for client distress and slow down to meet it where it is found.

As introduced in a previous chapter, CRT works with trauma via the Double ABC-X Model of family stress and resilience theory. This includes assessing the variables of stressors, resources, and perceptions of the situation, all contributing to the extent of trauma or crisis. This views adaptability as a key feature in resilience, both personally and relationally.

Therapeutic Considerations for Trauma

When working with trauma, clinicians must be mindful of the physical and psychological impacts throughout therapy:

1. If meeting in-person, set up the physical space to allow the client to have personal space and direct line-of-sight to the door. Ideally, the therapist won't be positioned between them and the exit. If meeting online, reiterate prioritization of their confidentiality and respecting their privacy.
2. Be sensitive to your nonverbals.
3. Be direct and concise in questions and reflections. If helpful, you may provide explanations of intention: *"If I say or ask something and you want to know why, please feel welcome to ask."*
4. The client's emotional regulation may be low, often hidden by high emotion suppression. Common emotions associated with religious trauma confusion, fear, anxiety, guilt, depression and sadness, anger.
5. Consistently ask for consent pertaining to questions and areas of conversation: *"Does it feel okay if we stay in this area of conversation for a while longer?"*, *"Is it okay to hover on this for a little bit?"* Give them permission to "come up for air," balancing discussing trauma and something less intense for them.
6. Consistently ask for consent before doing any kind of physical touch, both between yourself and the client and between members of the client system.
7. Pace of therapy may be slower due to fragility and uncertainty. We build on scaffolds of their strengths; we need those to be solid, so take time as needed on that foundation.
8. There may be a tendency in the person to respond with 'I don't know,' or to turn to others to provide answers for them. Normalize this and allow the client time to consider the possibilities, potentially benefiting from the reminder that there is not a right answer. This is, by itself, a therapeutic intervention.
9. With religious trauma, be careful with your language, as some common phrases are rooted in specific faiths ("This is your journey/testimony," "walk the straight and narrow," "it's a sign of the times," or "wash your hands" of someone).
10. As always, invite their feedback of what helps.

Trauma-Informed Assessment

Before diving into other assessment questions, prepare the client with language of empowerment: *"I'd like to learn more about you and your trauma. This process may be uncomfortable. If you don't feel comfortable or don't want to answer certain questions, that's completely okay."* This sets a precedence of request/giving permission or consent (and honoring if they say no). If they do not want to provide information about content, it is appropriate to ask if it is acceptable to talk about emotions about the topic, both now and at the time of the event(s). In addition to systemic and sex-therapy assessment questions, compassionate trauma-based questions include:

"How have you experienced situations and/or relationships that included abandonment? Betrayal? Humiliation? Injustice? Rejection?"
 What would you like me to know about those occasions? How frequent were they? How recently did they last occur? What's your relationship with the other people involved (how they are related, where and when they interact, feelings about that person)? How did you respond to those situations at the time? Have you told people these stories before? Who did you tell? How was it received? What's your relationship with those memories now?
 Assess for ongoing trauma sources. Is the client still at risk of abuse or neglect by their source, including a group (such as loved ones who are still members of a specific church)? Are there any reports that legally need to be made, such as child or adult protective services?

"What feelings or emotions do you typically tie with the idea of your trauma?"
 Thoughts? Behaviors? Where did you learn those?

"How did you learn what trauma is/was?"
 How old were you? What was happening in your life at that time? Who were the "big players" in that learning experience?

"How do you typically respond to times when you lack control, feel unsafe or distressed?"
 Do you tend more toward fight, flight, freeze, or something different? What has helped you cope with traumas so far? When was the last time you took those steps to get through a difficult moment?
 Assess for self-harm and substance use specifically; they are common maladaptive coping mechanisms, along with suicidality and homicidality.

"How do you feel in your body as we reflect on your experiences right now?"
 How does it feel to reflect on trauma as a relationship rather than an event? Assess for mind–body connection.

"What role does shame play in your life?"
How do you distinguish guilt and shame?

"To what extent are you preoccupied with being judged for your choices, by peers, leaders, or a higher power?"
What thoughts and emotions come with that concern? To what extent do others impact your perspectives or life decisions? What about sexual life decisions, specifically?

In addition to these questions, consider having questions about trauma in pre-session paperwork, giving a nonverbal space for the client to identify past trauma and indicate their degree of comfort verbally addressing it. This can be especially important with other people (family, partner[s], group members) present. There are also several trauma-focused assessment tools including the Brief Trauma Questionnaire (BTQ), the Trauma History Questionnaire (THQ), and the Life Stressor Checklist – Revised (LSC-R). For religious or spiritual trauma, there is the Spiritual Harm & Abuse Scale – Clinical Screener (SHAS-CS). Be aware, many of these are focused on the content of the painful memories and should not be required.

Intervention Applications with Trauma

As with previous chapters, let's identify specific examples of each of CRT's unique interventions as pertaining to trauma, sexual trauma, sexual self-expression, and building the ability to give and receive compassion for self and others.

Language Clarification

After trauma, redefining or distinguishing specific memories or ideas will be central to healing. This can be handily addressed through the Venn diagram version of the meaning-making intervention, having different circles represent different memories or meanings associated with terms or ideas. Finding spaces to replace "but" with "and" remains helpful to balance and validate conflicting thoughts and emotions tied to trauma experiences juxtaposed by personal values:

- Seeking to understand sexual expression can feel both scary/disconnecting *and* fulfilling/connecting.
- Sexual relationships and personal preferences can be both difficult *and* worthwhile to explore.
- Relationships with people and communities can be traumatizing *and* hold other emotions, including love.

Permission for *both* addresses the seeming disparity of loving someone who has hurt us – you can do both. This can be easily explored through parts language, which is commonly used in trauma processing therapy: Part of me has happy memories with the trauma source (person, place, or group); part of me has been very hurt by it. Both are valid. In trauma treatment with CRT, the part that therapy is addressing is the version of us that learned to survive the trauma. The clients now get to offer that part of them the love and advocacy that was denied previously through the abandonment, betrayal, humiliation, injustice, or rejection of the traumatic incidents. We are delineating vulnerability or softness from failure or weakness.

Compassionate Contextualization

Not all clients will connect their past trauma with current behavioral or cognitive response patterns. For many people, we acquire our beliefs and behavioral cues in contexts that consider these normal or helpful, such as house rules growing up. When the context is highly rigid or restrictive, exploring the impact of their influences can be like deprogramming after a cult. In CRT, we contextualize the client's relationship with the value system's, looking at the positive, negative, and neutral impact to them in the past and present:

o When were they taught this value? How was it reinforced?
o What is a positive memory they have associated with that system?
o When are times they felt a sense of belonging?
o When are times they felt safe, even overtly comforted or purposeful?
o When was an early time they remember questioning this value system? How did they manage or process that - Did they talk to anyone about it? How did they resolve this questioning? How does it feel to notice these and name them now?

The purpose is to normalize mixed feelings about experiences and why they may not have felt the extent of abuse at the time. It also serves to reiterate that we do not have to fall into a binary of something being good or evil; people and systems are too complex for such simplicity.

Next, apply "How does it make sense?" questions to recognize and validate specifically how these impact one's relationship with sexuality. Therapy can go through specific challenges a person has, including with their sexual identity or self-expression. Here are a few examples:

• "How does it make sense that biological or slang terms for sex organs create a physical discomfort in me?"

- "How does it make sense that specific sexual actions feel physically or emotionally uncomfortable to me, such as past experiences lacking consent or placing blame on me for the actions of others?"
- "How does it make sense that I have a difficult time distinguishing sex and gender, or nudity and sexual activity?"

All of these have very real answers worth reiterating to yourself to show compassion! As always, throughout this process, there is a perpetual opportunity for compassion. The client can ask and answer the question, "How does it make sense I haven't been compassionate about this before?" When working with trauma, it is also especially important to do the mindfulness steps of contextualizing, checking for current bodily awareness to stay in the present and asking what the person needs at the present moment.

For memories that are harder to speak aloud or more overtly abusive, not all information has to be verbally reviewed or shared. This process is about the client knowing the context, not the clinician. For others in the client system, it may be important to know there *is* history and then develop emotional safety leading up to the option, not requirement, to share more information and have it received compassionately.

Disentangling

Disentangling within trauma covers linear assumptions about people, including self, and sex. A few types of (incorrect!) assumptions in trauma are:

- Assumptions of intent resulting in future-telling or minimizing someone else's responsibility ("He's only flirting with me because he wants sex," or, "They didn't mean to hurt me, so I have to forgive them")
- Assumptions of personalization ("I'm at fault," "I must have wanted it since I got aroused," "I didn't do enough to stop it," in areas of limited or minimal control)

In response to these, the therapist can provide psychoeducation, such as normalizing arousal response to physical stimulation or the opposite, vaginal dryness or erectile dysfunction, which are often rooted in personal or relational insecurity or distress in the moment.

Similar to above, the therapist might ask, *"What else might someone think?"* or *"If you knew a stranger had the same thing happen, what might you think of them?"* With trusted loved ones, variations of the question could be, *"What would you hope someone else would think of you in that moment instead?"* or, *"What would it be like to take the pressure off yourself to know what they're thinking? To recognize, humanly, that it outside your capacity to read their mind?"*

Last, but not least, is the disentangling of meaning- making. As we've described in previous chapters, we are humbly asking, *"Would it be ok if I [the therapist] offered a different meaning I have heard about that idea?"*:

- What is the meaning of emotions, emotionality, and emotions' tie to sexual expression? (What if it is a method of honoring oneself, the human experience, and, debatably, one's higher power?)
- What is the meaning of trauma? Or what does it say about someone to have trauma or be traumatized by something? (Could it be a reason to intentionally and mindfully address a problem rather than a reason to avoid something?)
- Meaning of not fighting back during past occasions of abuse/trauma (What difference does it make to view this not as personal weakness or failure but instead as a survival instinct or simply not being aware at the time of the detriment potential because, at that time, in that moment, it seemed so normal?)

This is also a space to create new meaning of life and sexuality. As stated by a famed ACT theorist, "The antidote to insignificance and powerlessness is committed action: Operating within our locus of control. We focus on what we can do, what we can influence, what we can contribute through acting on our values" (Harris, 2021, p. 301).

Positive Restorations

Restorations about sex after trauma are positive healing statements. They are reminders of who you are, instead of who you are not. This can be permission to learn more about physical sex education, labels of sexual orientation, and balancing emotions around identifying outside the cis/heteronorm. All these can be disentangled individually or in conjunction with loved ones to further build emotional safety together and practice nonjudgmental curiosity.

In session, restorative conversations can explore when a partner responds to another from their traumatized part, particularly tied to sexual expression using a similar structure to what has previously been introduced:

1. Personally identify the painful past situation or memory (the abandonment, betrayal, humiliation, injustice, or rejection).
2. Identify what survival or connection effort you tried at the time.
3. Identify how it makes sense that it has historically been difficult to be compassionate to your past self or the person who contributed to the pain of the situation.

4. What underlying belief, value, or part of me is feeling unheard or uncared for? What does that part of me need right now?
5. Knowing what I know about my past self, how does it make sense that this is significant to them? How do I feel about that significance now?
6. What did that part of me need back then? How can I provide a version of that now?
7. What do I need right now to offer compassion and comfort to myself? (Complete this to the best of your ability independently)
8. What do I see/hear my loved ones need to feel compassionately loved right now?

In private spaces, such as at home, positive restorations can include restoring the relationship with one's body. This does not have to be sexual and uses nonjudgmental curiosity to allow for neutral, noninvasive interactions with one's body. For example, nonsexual touch or seeking personal anatomical understanding (familiarizing yourself with how your sexual organs look, feel, etc.) can allow a body to be explored outside imminent sexual purposes. This is a compassionate reiteration of the neutrality and goodness, not evilness, of the human body. When someone feels more comfortable with their own bodies, it can lead to more enjoyment of sexual touch and enjoyments, if a person chooses. This can incorporate aspects of Sensate Focus Therapy with nonjudgmental curiosity between partners regarding pace or interests.

Furthermore, individual personal check-ins can still be written activities. Clients may write letters to their past self or the loved one, or a part of someone still impacted by the traumatizing memory, expressing their compassion for that version of the person at the time. People can journal about the sexual self specifically and offer reflections to their loved one(s):

• What is something we (current and past self) did today that contributed to improving care for my body or soul, even a little bit or for a little while?
• What is something today for which I can offer the traumatized part (mine or my loved one's) some grace?
• How to I still hold hope for that part to feel better tomorrow?

Temporary Agreements

Particularly with sex and recovering from past trauma, this intervention is focused on a willingness to test the uncomfortable without crossing into what is painful. The goal remains for there to be mutual permission to self and trusted other(s) to try new things and say no to them after a trial period. In this case, that could be the question, *"If sex feels like a bad fit at this moment, what feels ok instead?"* This could be different types of physical touch, nonpenetrative sex, or other connecting activities. As the therapist, identify overlaps among individuals' answers and explore how this can feel different from rejection. From there, we can ask for the temporary terms, *"What would it be like to do that over the next few weeks?"*

Other versions of this that are tied to both sexual wellbeing and trauma are, *"How would you feel or act different if you believed you had innate worth and that your sexual self was a legitimate part of you?"* and, *"How would you like your sexual expression to be if you got to define it instead of the trauma getting to? What would you be doing differently?"* and for both, *"What would it be like to do one of those over the next few weeks, as if it was true?"*

Modality Comparison: Narrative Therapy

Narrative therapy is a popular choice to treat trauma because it emphasizes reauthoring, the redefining of trauma's impact on a person or relationship. There is also a version called narrative exposure therapy for complex trauma.

In both Narrative and CRT, the approach to trauma emphasizes empowering the client through resilience and amending one's role in the relationship with trauma – moving from victim versus survivor, being an agent of change. In both modalities, therapists lead change in the clients' emotional experiences of traumatic memories, not the memories themselves. A common method within this is externalization, which asserts "the problem is the problem," not the person. Therapy develops self-soothing responses to trauma triggers, like those based in senses or significance. The goal is not to avoid triggers but to be able to stay present when they happen, mindfully differentiating the current moment and interactions from those of the past.

However, CRT differs from narrative work in key ways. The latter leans on healing via the telling of a story, particularly factual events and the psychological perception of those at the time, rewriting those memories from a new perspective, and finding exceptions to damaging narratives. CRT focuses on healing through compassion for the you that experienced the event(s) and the innate internal goodness that was taken advantage of, such as the desire to love and be loved. CRT prioritizes decreasing shame on someone's past self and the decisions they made amidst the trauma, taking an appropriate amount of accountability, and eventually offering the love and support to themselves now that they needed at the time of the event.

Case Example

Let's hear from our case example. Sylvia and Dan have continued on in their sessions exploring the sexual messages they've received growing up, and exploring what their authentic erotic voices look like for each of them.

Therapist:	So it seems like for the two of you, we're really beginning to see the impact of the sexual messages you both received, and especially for you Dan.
Dan:	Yeah, it really feels like a huge piece of things for me. And there's something about that I wanted to bring up that I know has impacted me.
T:	Thanks so much for making that known, Dan. I'd love to hear about that. Sylvia, does that work for you?
Sylvia:	Yeah, I'd love to hear about this.
D:	So I know that for me, a huge piece of who I'm supposed to be as a sexual person came from what I heard in church. And I'm processing and really trying to accept that I'm not this dominant and intense sexual person. But I know that I still definitely feel like I'm wrong for that? And I know that a piece of this is the anal stuff. Like Sylvia wanted to try putting her finger in my ass one time because she thought it could be fun and when she did I really enjoyed it. And then immediately afterwards I felt so much shame for it because there was this part of me that was like "no this is wrong, and I'm wrong for liking it."
S:	Oh, Dan . . .
T:	Thank you for cueing us into that. First and foremost, that makes so much sense to me, and I think it takes a lot of courage to examine these narratives and piece them together. *(Compassionate validation)*
S:	Yeah, I mean I knew that there were things from your upbringing that were impactful, but I didn't realize how deeply they permeated into the sexual interactions. I remember that interaction we had though.
T:	Dan, correct me if I'm wrong, it seems like for you, based on religious messages you received growing up you learned that liking certain things or wanting certain things is "bad?"

D: Oh absolutely. Like sex was for procreation and just doing whatever you wanted was "giving into fleshly desire," which was bad. Sex was something that you reserved for marriage and then for having children, but it wasn't supposed to be this unhinged space where you did whatever you wanted.

T: So Dan, I'm hearing that for you when this happened with Sylvia it felt really enjoyable for you and there was a lot of sexual gratification that happened for you.

D: Without a doubt.

T: And it also seems like there was a shame response that happened afterwards because there was a part of you that learned experimenting and engaging in things like digital anal penetration was "wrong."

D: Yeah.

T: Sylvia, I want to hear from you a bit on this. What's coming up for you as we think about this?

S: I mean it makes a lot of sense to me right, like if you learn all your life that this thing is wrong or that you're not supposed to do something then of course if you do it you're gonna feel bad about it. I just wish that we could be who we want to be and I know that I feel frustrated when I feel like I'm continuously compromising. I want to make so much space for his emotional experience, and also know that it's hard for me.

T: I hear that Sylvia, absolutely. It definitely can feel frustrating to want to be your most authentic self, and it seems like that feels hard for you to do right now as well.

S: Yeah, I guess that's true. I hadn't thought about it like that.

T: I'm curious Dan, are there specific memories that come to mind for you that really reinforced some of these ideas?

D: Yeah, there definitely are. I mean there are overarching just messages in general, but I also remember this one youth camp I went to in high school and they split up boys and girls and talked to us about sex. And I remember them talking about all the things that were "bad" and then the things that were "good." And part of the "bad" things were doing things that made you a sodomite, so anal penetration or intercourse. I remember that even then I'd thought about trying different things and that was part of it and automatically was like "well, this means I'm damned." *(Positive restoration – identifying painful situation/memory)*

T: Oh wow Dan, thanks for bringing that forward. What an intense message to receive especially surrounding sex and sexual expression. It makes so much sense to me that you felt really impacted by that.

S: I can imagine that must have been hard to hear.

T: Thanks for making space for that Sylvia, and recognizing that for Dan. Beautifully done there. Dan, I'm wondering, how would your life be different if you believed that your sexual self was a legitimate part of you?

D: Oh wow, I'd probably feel like I could do things like that without being sent to hell for it.

T: I can imagine it might feel different and maybe create space for you to feel more free? What do you think?

D: Oh yeah, I mean if I didn't have that thought I'd feel like I could do whatever I wanted honestly.

T: That makes sense. I'm curious, there's no pressure with this but let's just imagine for a minute, what would it be like to do one of those things over the next few weeks, as if it was true that your sexual self was legitimate, and beautiful? *(Introducing potential temporary agreement)*

D: Oh, I think being able to do that would be amazing. I want to be able to not have these narratives in my mind and want to be able to do things differently. I just know I'm not there yet.

T: Absolutely, we want to approach things in a pace that feels good for us. I love that we were just able to entertain that idea for a moment and gently explore what that might look and feel like for us. *(Use of "we" language)*

References

Aguilar-Raab, C., Jarczok, M. N., Warth, M., Stoffel, M., Winter, F., Tieck, M., Berg, J., Negi, L. T., Harrison, T., Pace, T. W. W., & Ditzen, B. (2018). Enhancing social interaction in depression (SIDE study): Protocol of a randomised controlled trial on the effects of a cognitively based compassion training (CBCT) for couples. *BMJ Open, 8*. https://bmjopen.bmj.com/content/8/9/e020448

Allender, D. (Host). (2014, Dec. 14). Defining Trauma and Abuse. In *Allender Center at the Seattle School* [audio podcast episode]. https://theallendercenter.org/2014/12/allender-center-podcast-defining-trauma-abuse/

American Psychiatric Association (2022). *Diagnostic and statistical manual of mental disorders*, 5th ed, text revision (DSM-5-TR). American Psychiatric Association, Washington, DC.

Aminzadeh, M. S., & Bolghan-Abadi, M. (2022). Effectiveness of the compassion-focused therapy on self-criticism and marital intimacy among couples. *International Journal of Body, Mind, and Culture, 9*(4), 335–342. http://dx.doi.org/10.22122/ijbmc.v9i4.395

Ash, M., Harrison, T., Pinto, M., DiClemente, R., & Negi, L.T. (2021). A model for cognitively-based compassion training: theoretical underpinnings and proposed mechanisms. *Social Theory Health, 19*(1), 43–67. https://doi.org/10.1057/s41285-019-00124-x.B

Attachment Project (2020). *What is ethical non-monogamy? Intro to ENM relationships.* www.attachmentproject.com/enm/

Baldwin, S., Bandarian-Balooch, S., & Adams, R. (2020). Attachment and compassion-threat: Influence of a secure attachment-prime. *Psychology and Psychotherapy: Theory, Research and Practice, 93*(3), 520–536. https://doi.org/10.1111/papt.12244

Barnard, L. K., & Curry, J. F. (2011). Self-compassion: Conceptualizations, correlates, & interventions. *Review of General Psychology, 15*(4), 289–303. https://doi.org/10.1037/a0025754

Barth, J., Bermetz, L., Heim, E., Trelle, S., & Tonia, T. (2013). The current prevalence of child sexual abuse worldwide: A systematic review and meta-analysis. *International Journal of Public Health, 58*(3), 469–483. https://doi.org/10.1007/s00038-012-0426-1

Birch, P., & Braun-Harvey, D. (2019). Sexual health principles and the procurement of sexual services: Evidence of the interface between sexual health and criminal justice. *Journal of Forensic Practice, 21*(2), 145–157. https://doi.org/10.1108/JFP-02-2019-0006

Bell, T., Dixon, A., & Kolts, R. (2017). Developing a compassionate internal supervisor: Compassion-focused therapy for trainee therapists. *Clinical Psychology and Psychotherapy, 24*, 632–648. https://doi.org/10.1002/cpp.2031

Bloom, P. (2017). *Against empathy: The case for rational compassion.* Random House.

Bolt, O.C., Jones, F.W., Rudaz, M., Ledermann, T., & Irons, C. (2019). Self-compassion and compassion towards one's partner mediate the negative association between insecure attachment and relationship quality. *Journal of Relationships Research 10*(e20), 1–9. https://doi.org/10.1017/jrr.2019.17

Bourbeau, L. (2020). *Heal your wounds & find your true self.* Editions E.T.C. Inc.

Bradshaw, J. (2017). *Healing the shame that binds you.* Health Communications.

Brown, B. (2015). *Daring greatly: How the courage to be vulnerable transforms the way we live, love, parent, and lead.* Avery Publishing.

Campbell, J. C., & Christopher, J. C. (2012). Teaching mindfulness to create effective counselors. *Journal of Mental Health Counseling, 34*(3), 213–226. https://doi.org/10.17744/mehc.34.3.j756585201572581

Carnes, P. J. (2001). *Out of the shadows: Understanding sexual addiction*, 3rd edition. Hazelden.

Dailey, D. (1997). The failure of sexuality education: Meeting the challenge of behavioral change in a sex-positive context. In: J. Maddock (Ed.) *Sexuality Education in Postsecondary and Professional Training Settings* (pp. 87–97). Hawthorne Press.

Dayle, J. (2025). *People-pleaser versus people manager.* Beyond Codependency. www.jennadayle.com/blog/people-pleaser-vs-people-manager

Dayle, J. (@beyondcodependency) (n.d.) Range of codependency. Instagram. Retrieved January 31, 2025, from www.instagram.com/beyondcodependency/ and www.jennadayle.com/

Edwards, C., Allan, R., Marzo, N., Wynfield, T., & Hicks, R. (2023). The use of emotionally focused therapy with polyamorous relationships. *Family Process, 62*, 1362–1376. https://doi.org/10.1111/famp.12934

Ellis, H. M., Hook, J. N., Zuniga, S., Hodge, A. S., Ford, K. M., Davis, D. E., & Van Tongeren, D. R. (2022). Religious/spiritual abuse and trauma: A systematic review of the empirical literature. *Spirituality in Clinical Practice, 9*(4), 213–231. https://doi.org/10.1037/scp0000301

Erekson, D. M., Griner, D., & Beecher, M. E. (2024). Compassion focused therapy for groups: Transdiagnostic treatment for turbulent times. *International Journal of Group Psychotherapy, 74*(2), pp. 149–176. https://doi.org/10.1080/0020728 4.2024.2314278

Fern, J. (2020). *Polysecure.* Thorntree Press.

Francis, C. A. (2023). The new stages of grief. Mindfulness Meditation Institute. https://mindfulnessmeditationinstitute.org/2023/02/16/the-new-stages-of-grief/

Giordano, A. L., Schmit, M. K., Clement, K., Potts, E. E., & Graham, A. R. (2022). Pornography use and sexting trends among American adolescents: Data to inform school counseling programming and practice. *Professional School Counseling, 26*(1). https://doi.org/10.1177/2156759X221137287

Gilbert, P., & Simos, G. (Eds.) (2022). *Compassion focused therapy: Clinical practice and applications.* Routledge.

Glover Tawwab, N. (2023). *Setting boundaries: Excerpts from The Boundaries Flip Chart.* Pesi Publishing, Inc., therapist.com. https://6951996.fs1.hubs potusercontent-na1.net/hubfs/6951996/therapist.com/Squeeze%20Page%20 Assets/Boundary%20Setting%20Guide.pdf

Goerlich, S. (2023). *With sprinkles on top: Everything vanilla people and their kinky partners need to know to communicate, explore, and connect.* Sounds True Publishing.

Gregory, A. (2014). The impact of trauma on sexual functioning. *International Journal of Urological Nursing, 8*(1), 44–48. https://doi.org/10.1111/ijun.12031

Haghighifard, S., Khaleghipour, S., & Zarneyestanak, M. (2023). Effectiveness of compassion-focused positive couple therapy on entitlement schema, bullying, and marital adjustment in narcissistic men. *Journal of Psychological Studies, 19*(2), 16. https://psychstudies.alzahra.ac.ir/article_7291.html

Harris, R. (2021). *Trauma-focused ACT: A practitioner's guide to working with mind, body, and emotion using acceptance & commitment therapy.* Context Press.

Ho, P. S. Y. (2006). The (charmed) circle game: Reflections on sexual hierarchy through multiplesexual relationships. *Sexualities, 9*(5), 547–564. https://doi.org/10.1177/1363460706069966

Holt-Lunstad, J., & Smith, T.B. (2012). *Social relationships and mortality, 6*(1), 41–53. https://doi.org/10.1111/j.1751-9004.2011.00406.x

Huppmann, R. H. (2014). *Overcoming sexual dependency: Using accelerated experiential dynamic psychotherapy (AEDP) to heal attachment wounds.* [Unpublished master thesis]. St. Stephen's College. https://doi.org/10.7939/R3G44J48C

Jennings, T. R. (2024). *Codependency: What it is and how to break free.* Come and Reason Ministries. https://comeandreason.com/codependency-what-it-is-and-how-to-break-free/

Jiménez, L., Hidalgo, V., Baena, S., León, A., & Lorence, B. (2019). Effectiveness of structural-strategic family therapy in the treatment of adolescents with mental health problems and their families. *International Journal of Environmental Research and Public Health, 16*(7), 1255–1269. https://doi.org/10.3390/ijerph16071255

Karris, M., & Caldwell, B. E. (2015). Integrating emotionally focused therapy, self-compassion, and compassion-focused therapy to assist shame-prone couples who have experienced trauma. *The Family Journal, 23*(4), 346–357. https://doi-org.acu.idm.oclc.org/10.1177/1066480715601676

Kauppi, M. (2020). *Polyamory: A clinical toolkit for therapists (and their clients).* Rowman and Littlefield.

Kelly, L. C., Spencer, C. M., Keilholtz, B., McAllister, P., & Stith, S. M. (2022). Is separate the new equal? A meta-analytic review of correlates of intimate partner violence victimization for black and white women in the United States. *Family Process, 61*(4), 1473–1488. https://doi.org/10.1111/famp.12754

Kemper, D. (Writer), & Scheerer, R. (1989, July 10). Peak performance (Season 2, Episode 21) [TV series episode]. In R. Berman, M. Hurley, & Roddenberry, G. (Executive Producers), *Star Trek: The Next Generation.* Paramount Productions.

Kuncewicz, D., Lachowicz-Tabaczek, K., & Załuski, J. (2014). Why insight in psychotherapy does not always lead to behaviour change? *Polish Journal of Applied Psychology, 12*(2). http://archive.sciendo.com/PJAP/pjap.2014.12.issue-2/pjap-2015-0011/pjap-2015-0011.pdf

Leary, M. R., Tate, E. B., Adams, C. E., Allen, A. B., & Hancock, J. (2007). Self-compassion and reactions to unpleasant self-relevant events: The implications of treating oneself kindly. *Journal of Personality and Social Psychology, 92*, 887–904. https://doi.org/10.1037/0022-3514.92.5.887

Leaviss, J., & Uttley, L. (2015). Psychotherapeutic benefits of compassion-focused therapy: An early systematic review. *Psychological Medicine, 45*, 927–945. https://pmc.ncbi.nlm.nih.gov/articles/PMC4413786/pdf/S0033291714002141a.pdf

Lindsay, E. K., & Creswell, J. D. (2014). Helping the self help others: Self-affirmation increases self-compassion and pro-social behaviors. *Frontiers in Psychology*, *5*, 421–430. https://doi.org/10.3389/fpsyg.2014.00421

Lindgren, J., Winston, D., & Sotelo Matlack, E. (Hosts) (2017). "R.A.D.A.R." *Multiamory* [Audio podcast]. https://static1.squarespace.com/static/54e132a8e4b0be 2d4c9300a7/t/5a1cef7371c10b644b09d61d/1511845752513/Multiamory+ RADAR+Template.pdf

Lord, S. A. (2017). Mindfulness and spirituality in couple therapy: The use of meditative dialogue to help couples develop compassion and empathy for themselves and each other. *Australian and New Zealand Journal of Family Therapy*, *38*(1), 98–114. https://doi.org/10.1002/anzf.1201

Luberto, C. M., Shinday, N., Song, R., Philpotts, L. L., Park, E. R., Fricchione, G. L., & Yeh, G. Y. (2018). A systematic review and meta-analysis of the effects of meditation on empathy, compassion, and prosocial behaviors. *Mindfulness*, *9*(3), 708–724. https://pmc.ncbi.nlm.nih.gov/articles/PMC6081743/pdf/ nihms914995.pdf

McCubbin, H. I., & Patterson, J. M. (1983a). Family stress and adaptation to crises: A Double ABCX Model of family behavior. In D. H. Olson & R. C. Miller (Eds.), *Family studies review yearbook (vol. 1)* (pp. 87–106). Beverly Hills, CA: Sage.

McCubbin, H. I., & Patterson, J. M. (1983b). The family stress process: The Double ABCX Model of family adjustment and adaptation. In H. I. McCubbin, M. Sussman, & J. M. Patterson (Eds.), *Social stress and the family: Advances and developments in family stress theory and research* (pp. 7–37). New York: Haworth.

McNamee, S., Rasera, E. F., & Martins, P. (2023). *Practicing therapy as social construction*. Sage.

Millard, L. A., Wan, M. W., Smith, D. M., & Wittkowski, A. (2023). The effectiveness of compassion focused therapy with clinical populations: A systematic review and meta-analysis. *Journal of Affective Disorders*, *326*, 168–192. https:// doi.org/10.1016/j.jad.2023.01.010

Moral-Jiménez, M. d.l.V., & Mena-Baumann, A. (2024). Emotional dependence and narcissism in couple relationships: Echo and Narcissus syndrome. *Behavioral Sciences*, *14*(12), 1190–1204. https://doi.org/10.3390/bs14121190

Nagoski, E. (2015). *Come as you are*. Simon & Schuster.

Nagoski, E. (2024). *Come together: The science (and art!) of creating lasting sexual connections*. Ballantine Books.

Neff, K. D. (2003). The development and validation of a scale to measure self-compassion. *Self and Identity*, *2*(3), 223–250. https://self-compassion.org/ wp-content/uploads/publications/empirical.article.pdf

Neff, K. D. (2015). The five myths of self-compassion. *Psychotherapynetworker. org*, *47*, 31–35. https://self-compassion.org/wp-content/uploads/2019/03/The_5_ Myths_of_Self-Compassion-Psychotherapy-Networker.pdf

Neff, K. D. (2023). Self-compassion: Theory, method, research, and intervention. *Annual Review of Psychology*, *74*, 193–218. https://doi.org/10.1146/annurev- psych-032420-031047

Neff, K. D., & Germer, C. (2013). A pilot study and randomized controlled trial of the mindful self-compassion program. *Journal of Social and Clinical Psychology*, *69*(1), 28–44. https://doi.org/10.1002/jclp.21923

Neff, K. D., & McGehee, P. (2010). Self-compassion and psychological resilience among adolescents and young adults. *Self and Identity*, *9*(3), 225–240. https:// doi.org/10.1080/15298860902979307

Neff, K. D., & Vonk, R. (2009). Self-compassion versus global self-esteem: Two different ways of relating to oneself. *Journal of Personality, 77*, 23–50. https://doi.org/10.1111/j.1467-6494.2008.00537.x

Newman, B., & Newman, P. R. (2018). *Development through life: A psychosocial approach*, 13th edition. Wadsworth Publishing.

Olson, D. H., & Gorall, D. M. (2010). *FACES-IV manual*. Life Innovations. https://pedpsych.org/wp-content/uploads/2016/02/3_innovations.pdf

Ott, K. (2016). Sex and candy: Unwrapping how we define sexuality. *American Journal of Sexuality Education, 11*(1), 106–112. https://doi.org/10.1080/15546 128.2016.1146185

Panchuk, M. (2018). The shattered spiritual self: A philosophical exploration of religious trauma. *Res Philosophica, 95*(3), 505–530. https://doi.org/10.11612/resphil.1684

Panos, P. T., Jackson, J. W., Hasan, O., & Panos, A. (2014). Meta-analysis and systematic review assessing the efficacy of dialectical behavior therapy (DBT). *Research on Social Work ractice, 24*(2), 213–223. https://doi.org/10.1177/1049731513503047

Perel, E. (2017). *The state of affairs: Rethinking infidelity*. Harper Publications.

Pérez-Fuentes, G., Olfson, M., Villegas, L., Morcillo, C., Wang, S., & Blanco, D. (2013). Prevalence and correlates of child sexual abuse: A national study. *Comprehensive Psychiatry, 54*(1), 16–27. https://doi.org/10.1016/j.comppsych.2012.05.010

Petrocchi, N., Ottaviani, C., Cheli, S., Matos, M., Baldi, B., Basran, J. K., & Gilbert, P. (2024). The impact of compassion-focused therapy on positive and negative mental health outcomes: Results of a series of meta-analyses. *Clinical Psychology: Science and Practice, 31*(2), 230–247. https://doi.org/10.1037/cps0000193

Reach Beyond Domestic Violence. (2017). *Six different types of abuse*. https://reachma.org/blog/6-different-types-of-abuse/

Reynolds, V. (2013). "Leaning in" as imperfect allies in community work. *Conflict and Narrative: Explorations in Theory and Practice, 1*(1), pp. 53–75. http://journals.gmu.edu/NandC/issue/1

Rosenberg, R. (2015). *Continuum of self, Adapted from the human magnet syndrome emotional manipulators and codependents: Understanding the attraction*. Human Magnet Syndrome. https://maritalintimacyinst.com/wp-content/uploads/Codependency-and-the-Continuum-of-Self.pdf

Silva, C., Moreira, P., Moreira, D. S., Rafael, F., Rodrigues, A., Leite, A., Lopes, S., & Moreira, D. (2024). Impacts of adverse childhood experiences in young adults and adults: A systematic literature review. *Pediatric Reports, 16*, 461–481. https://doi.org/10.3390/pediatric16020040

Smith, S. G., Zhang, X., Basile, K. C., Merrick, M. T., Wang, J., Kresnow, M., & Chen, J. (2018). *The national intimate partner and sexual violence survey: 2015 data brief, updated release*. National Center for Injury Prevention and Control (U.S.), Division of Violence Prevention. https://stacks.cdc.gov/view/cdc/60893

Sullivan, K. (2018, Spring). Structure of codependency and its relationship to narcissism. *Journal of Heart Centered Therapies, 21*(1), 53–68. link.gale.com/apps/doc/A539922311/HRCA?u=txshracd2478&sid=bookmark-HRCA&xid=73ce7ed7.

Suppes, B. (2022). *Family systems theory simplified: Applying and understanding systemic therapy models*. Routledge.

Turner, G. W. (2020). The circles of sexuality: Promoting a strengths-based model within social work that provides a holistic framework for client sexual well-being.

In A.N. Mendenhall (Ed.), *Rooted in Strengths: Celebrating the Strengths Perspective in Social Work* (pp. 305–325), University of Kansas Libraries.

Victims of sexual violence: Statistics. Rape, Abuse, and Incest National Network (RAINN). https://rainn.org/statistics/victims-sexual-violence

Vosper, J., Irons, C., Mackenzie-White, K., Saunders, F., Lewis, R., & Gibson, S. (2023). Introducing compassion focused psychosexual therapy. *Sexual and Relationship Therapy, 38*(3), 320–352. https://doi.org/10.1080/14681994.2021.1902495

Weissman, A. S. (2024). *Compassion-focused parent therapy.* Child & Family Institute. https://childfamilyinstitute.com/factsheets/compassionate-parent-training/

Werner, K. H., Jazaieri, H., Goldin, P. R., Ziv, M., Heimberg, R. G., & Gross, J. J. (2012). Self-compassion and social anxiety disorder. *Anxiety, Distress, and Coping, 25*(5), 543–558. https://doi.org/10.1080/10615806.2011.608842

Worthington Jr, E. L., O'Connor, L. E., Berry, J. W., Sharp, C., Murray, R., & Yi, E. (2004). Compassion and forgiveness. In P. Gilbert (Ed.), *Compassion: Conceptualisations, research and use in psychotherapy* (pp. 168–169). Routledge, Taylor & Francis Group.

Wright, N. P., Turkington, D., Kelly, O. P., Davies, D., Jacobs, A. M., & Hopton, J. (2014). *Treating psychosis: A clinician's guide to integrating acceptance and commitment therapy, compassion-focused therapy, and mindfulness approaches within cognitive behavioral therapy tradition.* New Harbinger Publications, Inc.

Index

For Product Safety Concerns and Information please contact our EU
representative GPSR@taylorandfrancis.com
Taylor & Francis Verlag GmbH, Kaufingerstraße 24, 80331 München, Germany

www.ingramcontent.com/pod-product-compliance
Lightning Source LLC
Chambersburg PA
CBHW050349270326
41926CB00016B/3666

9 781032 848914